GENETICS
for dermatologists

The REMEDICA Genetics for... Series

Genetics for Cardiologists
Genetics for Dermatologists
Genetics for Haematologists

Coming soon

Genetics for Endocrinologists
Genetics for Oncologists
Genetics for Ophthalmologists
Genetics for Rheumatologists

Published by REMEDICA Publishing Limited
32-38 Osnaburgh Street, London, NW1 3ND, UK

Tel: +44 207 388 7677
Fax: +44 207 388 7678
Email: info@remedica.com
www.remedica.com

ISBN 1 901346 10 2
British Library Cataloguing-in-Publication Data
A catalogue record for this book is available from the British Library.

GENETICS
for dermatologists

The molecular genetic basis of dermatological disorders

Sherri J Bale
Clinical Director
GeneDx Inc

Series Editor:
Eli Hatchwell
Visiting Scientist
Cold Spring Harbor Laboratory

ReMEDICA*PUBLISHING*

Introduction to Genetics for… series

Medicine is changing. The revolution in molecular genetics has fundamentally altered our notions of disease aetiology and classification, and promises novel therapeutic interventions. Standard diagnostic approaches to disease focused entirely on clinical features and relatively crude clinical diagnostic tests. Little account was traditionally taken of possible familial influences in disease.

The rapidity of the genetics revolution has left many physicians behind, particularly those whose medical education largely preceded its birth. Even for those who might have been aware of molecular genetics and its possible impact, the field was often viewed as highly specialist and not necessarily relevant to everyday clinical practice. Furthermore, while genetic disorders were viewed as representing a small minority of the total clinical load, it is now becoming clear that the opposite is true: few clinical conditions are totally without some genetic influence.

The physician will soon need to be as familiar with genetic testing as he/she is with routine haematology and biochemistry analysis. While rapid and routine testing in molecular genetics is still an evolving field, in many situations such tests are already routine and represent essential adjuncts to clinical diagnosis (a good example is cystic fibrosis).

This series of monographs is intended to bring specialists up to date in molecular genetics, both generally and also in very specific ways that are relevant to the given speciality. The aims are generally twofold:

(i) to set the relevant speciality in the context of the new genetics in general and more specifically

(ii) to allow the specialist, with little experience of genetics or its nomenclature, an entry into the world of genetic testing as it pertains to his/her speciality

These monographs are not intended as comprehensive accounts of each speciality — such reference texts are already available. Emphasis has been placed on those disorders with a strong genetic aetiology and, in particular, those for which diagnostic testing is available.

The glossary is designed as a general introduction to molecular genetics and its language.

The revolution in genetics has been paralleled in recent years by the information revolution. The two complement each other, and the World Wide Web is a rich source of information about genetics. The following sites are highly recommended as sources of information:

1. PubMed. Free on-line database of medical literature.
   http://www.ncbi.nlm.nih.gov/PubMed/
2. NCBI. Main entry to genome databases and other information about the human genome project.
   http://www.ncbi.nlm.nih.gov/
3. OMIM. On line inheritance in Man. The On-line version of McKusick's catalogue of Mendelian Disorders. Excellent links to PubMed and other databases.
   http://www.ncbi.nlm.nih.gov/omim/
4. Mutation database, Cardiff.
   http://www.uwcm.ac.uk/uwcm/mg/hgmd0.html

Eli Hatchwell
Cold Spring Harbor Laboratory

July 2000

Preface

While the genetic revolution begun two decades ago was being waged in the arenas of Mendelian disorders predisposing to cancer, neurological and haematological diseases, and inborn errors of metabolism, among others, the field of genetics in dermatology lay fallow. It was not until 1991, when Dr Ervin Epstein discovered that a mutation in either the gene for keratin 5 or keratin 14 could cause epidermolysis bullosa simplex, that the field of dermatology finally became a player in the new game of genetics. Since then, the genetic basis of many hereditary dermatological disorders has been identified. As is usual, the disorders that follow strict Mendelian inheritance patterns have been the first to reveal their colours. Many of these genodermatoses are rare; most dermatologists will go their entire career seeing only one patient with a particular diagnosis. However, the information gained through investigations of the genetics of these experiments of nature has contributed tremendously to our understanding of the development and differentiation of the skin, and may eventually lead to new treatments and perhaps even cures. But of more immediate relevance for the patients and their families is that, in many cases, the information is now available to provide definitive diagnosis, genetic counselling, carrier detection and pre-natal diagnosis. The patients and families affected by these diseases deserve to be offered the benefits of this research, both for humanitarian reasons and for the fact that without their unselfish participation in the research these important discoveries would never have been made.

This book attempts to bring the information on those genodermatoses for which the molecular basis has been defined as of March, 2000, together in one easy-to-use volume. It is different from all the other books available on hereditary skin disease, in that it offers short, concise reviews of the state of knowledge about the molecular basis of the disease, unavailable in one place elsewhere. But this book is not several other things. *Genetics for Dermatologists* is not an encyclopaedia of hereditary skin disorders. For that, one must use the very best book in that class, *Genetic Skin Disorders* by Virginia P Sybert. Due to the nature of genetics research and the time to publication for books, *Genetics for Dermatologists* can only provide information up to the minute that the volume goes to press. By the time it is available for purchase there will likely be other genetic skin disorders where the molecular basis has been uncovered. Therefore, the reader is referred to the Online Mendelian Inheritance in Man, OMIM, which can be found on the World Wide Web at http://www.ncbi.nlm.nih.gov/omim/, and is supported by the Center for Medical Genetics, Johns Hopkins University (Baltimore, MD) and the National Center for Biotechnology Information, National Library of Medicine (Bethesda, MD). This web site will provide a brief summary of recent publications pertaining to the genetics of any hereditary disorder, and should be in the bookmark file of all dermatologists' and geneticists' web browser.

It is my hope that this volume will prove useful to the practitioner, and that regular updates will be forthcoming to enable interested dermatologists to provide the best care to their patients.

How to use this book

Each entry in this volume represents a disorder for which the molecular basis is relatively well defined, although in a few cases I have included a disorder where the relevant information is likely to be available within a year or so of publication of this book. If a patient with a genodermatosis presents in your office, a quick look in *Genetics for Dermatologists* will show whether the molecular basis has been defined. If the gene has been identified, the patient should be referred to a geneticist for counselling. Either yourself, or a genetics counsellor, can search the GeneTests database (http://www.genetests.org/) to determine whether clinical testing is available for molecular diagnosis and carrier detection in family members, and whether options exist for pre-natal diagnosis of the disease in the offspring of your patient. GeneTests will show which laboratories are offering these services, what tissue (blood, skin, cheek cells) is needed for diagnosis, how to collect and ship samples, and sometimes also the cost and turn-around time for results. If no labs are identified you can contact me at GeneDx, Inc. (sherrib@genedx.com).

Once a clinical diagnosis of a genodermatosis is made, it is important to guide the patient to appropriate support groups. The National Organization for Rare Disorders is the clearinghouse for such groups, and its home page can be found at [http://www.rarediseases.org/].

This volume does not provide detailed clinical information about each disorder, which can be found in several excellent books, including Virginia Sybert's *Genetic Skin Disorders* (1997). The most recent published research on virtually any hereditary disorder can be found by searching the Online Mendelian Inheritance in Man [http://www.ncbi.nlm.nih.gov/omim/].

Acknowledgements

I am indebted to Jorge Toro who provided moral support, brought several important articles to my attention, and most of all allowed me to use many of his personal collection of clinical photographs for this volume, which Harry Schaefer then prepared expertly for publication. My business partner and expert molecular biologist John Compton reviewed the *Diagnosis* section of each entry. I am grateful to many of my friends in the genetics and dermatology community who reviewed those entries that were in their areas of expertise, including John DiGiovanna (who read the whole book), Gabriele Richard, Ken Kraemer, Bill Gahl, Bill Rizzo, Laura Russell, Margaret Tucker, Dilys Parry, Larry Charnas and Alain Colige. I am particularly indebted to Virginia Sybert, without whose wonderful text on genetic skin disease I would not have known where to start *this* book. I also referred to *Epidermolysis Bullosa*, edited by Jo-David Fine et al., and *Dermatology in General Practice*, edited by T Fitzpatrick *et al.*

Finally, the patience of my husband Eric and of my children Nathan and Viktoria is greatly appreciated, as much time and attention that would have gone to them had to be re-focussed during the past year as I wrote this book.

Contents

1. Disorders of Cornification

Epidermolytic Hyperkeratosis

AKA

Bullous congenital ichthyosiform erythroderma; bullous erythroderma ichthyosiform congenita of Brocq; EHK

MIM

113800

Clinical features

Presents at birth with erythroderma and blisters. Hyperkeratosis develops over time. Palms and soles may be involved or completely spared. Patients often have a peculiar, sour odour.

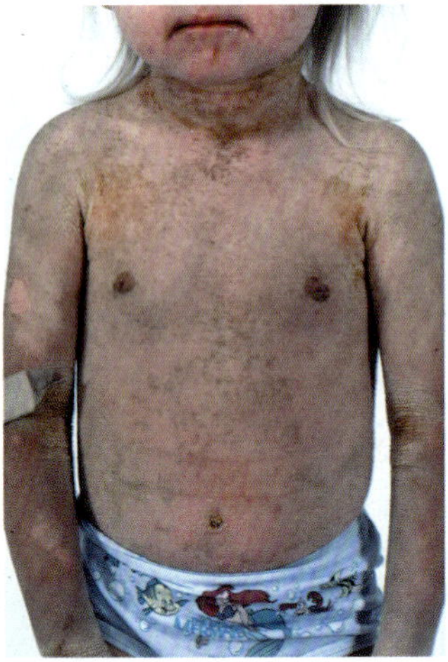

Epidermolytic hyperkeratosis in a young child.

Age of onset

Congenital

Epidemiology

1:300,000

Inheritance

Autosomal dominant; approximately 50% of cases are due to new mutational events

Chromosomal location

17q12-q21; 12q11-13

Genes

Mutations in either of the two supra-basal expressed keratins can cause EHK. KRT1, on chromosome 12, codes for keratin 1 (a type II keratin), and KRT10 (a type I keratin), on chromosome 17, codes for keratin 10. The keratin 1 and 10 proteins form heteroduplexes and higher-order complexes that generate an intermediate filament network to give the keratinocyte mechanical integrity. The keratin genes contain 7 or 8 exons (type I and II, respectively) in approximately 5-8 kb of genomic DNA.

Mutational spectrum

Most mutations affect the residues at the ends of the rod domains of the keratin proteins. The vast majority of mutations are single base changes leading to amino acid substitutions in the resultant keratin protein.

Effect of mutation

The presence of 50% abnormal keratin protein in the cell interferes with the assembly of normal intermediate size keratin filaments and causes the keratinocyte to become fragile.

Diagnosis

Epidermolytic hyperkeratosis of the supra-basal layers of the skin, especially the spinous layer, is observed on haemotoxylin- and eosin-stained fixed tissue obtained by biopsy. Direct sequencing of genomic DNA can identify the responsible mutation.

Counselling issues

The risk to offspring of affected individuals is 50%. Although most situations in which two unaffected parents have an affected child is due to a new mutational event in a germ cell or the embryo, there are very rare instances where unaffected parents have produced more than one child with EHK. In such a case, it is likely that one or the other parent has mosaicism of the germ line, and the risk to future offspring is 50%.

Linear Epidermolytic Naevus

AKA

Epidermolytic naevus syndrome; mosaic epidermolytic hyperkeratosis

MIM

163200

Clinical features

Raised, often verrucous or erythematous papules and plaques following lines of Blaschko. The lesions can be very extensive, or limited to a single papule.

Age of onset

Congenital, but can progress over time

Inheritance

Sporadic, due to somatic mutation

Genes

In many cases a mutation of KRT1 (chromosome 12) or KRT10 (chromosome 10) can be identified; however, depending on the extent of involvement, mutation identification can be difficult as only a small percentage of cells may carry the mutation.

Mutational spectrum

Most mutations affect the residues at the ends of the rod domains of the keratin proteins. The vast majority of mutations are single base changes leading to amino acid substitutions in the resultant keratin protein.

Diagnosis

EHK of the supra-basal layers of the skin, especially the spinous layer, is observed on haemotoxylin- and eosin-stained fixed tissue obtained by biopsy. It is frequently necessary to analyse DNA obtained from several tissue types to identify the mutation. Genomic DNA may have to be sequenced from blood as well as both involved and uninvolved skin.

Counselling issues

If the embryonic cells that eventually give rise to the germ cells carry the keratin mutation, the risk of passing the mutation to offspring is as high as 50%. In the case of such children, their disease will be the generalized form of EHK. The risk of recurrence to siblings of affected individuals is extremely low.

Ichthyosis Bullosa of Siemens

AKA

IBS

MIM

146800

Clinical features

Non-erythrodermic skin with generalized hyperkeratosis of variable severity, especially overlying the joints. The skin exhibits a Mauserung phenomenon — a superficial peeling of the stratum corneum.

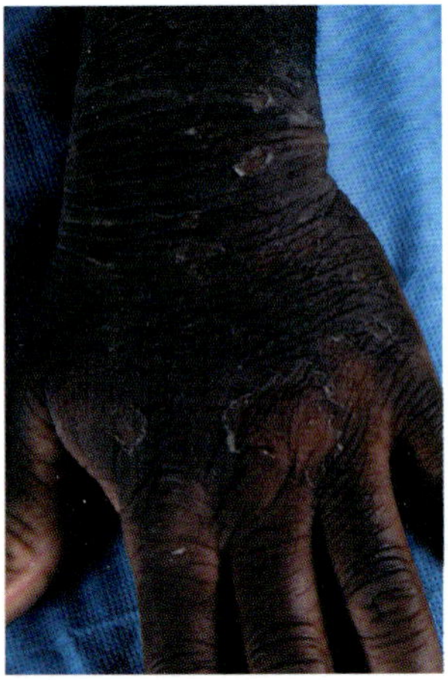

"Mauserung" phenomenon in ichthyosis bullosa of Siemens.

Age of onset

Blistering after minor trauma develops in infancy. The hyperkeratosis progresses over time.

Inheritance

Autosomal dominant

Chromosomal location

12q11-13

Gene

KRT2e, coding for the keratin protein 2e, a type II keratin gene, expressed in the upper spinous and granular layers of the skin. The expression partner of keratin 2e, if there is one, has not been determined.

Mutational spectrum

Mutations affect the rod domains of the keratin protein as in other keratin diseases, e.g. EHK and epidermolysis bullosa simplex. Missense mutations are observed, especially affecting Glu^{493}, as well as other residues in the region.

Diagnosis

EHK is observed in the upper spinous and granular layers of the skin on microscopic examination. Mutations in KRT2e can be identified by direct sequence analysis of genomic DNA.

Counselling issues

This disorder is usually milder, with respect to skin fragility and hyperkeratosis, than EHK, although there are exceptions. Mutation analysis of all three keratins, KRT1, KRT10 and KRT2e, should be performed.

Lamellar Ichthyosis

AKA

Non-erythrodermic lamellar ichthyosis; ichthyosis congenita type II

MIM

242300

Clinical features

Collodion membrane present at birth. Once membrane is shed, brown plate-like scales develop during infancy and involve the entire integument. Ectropion and eclabium, and scarring alopecia are frequent features. Palms and soles may be severely involved with thick hyperkeratosis. Hypohidrosis leads to heat intolerance. Milder phenotypes also occur.

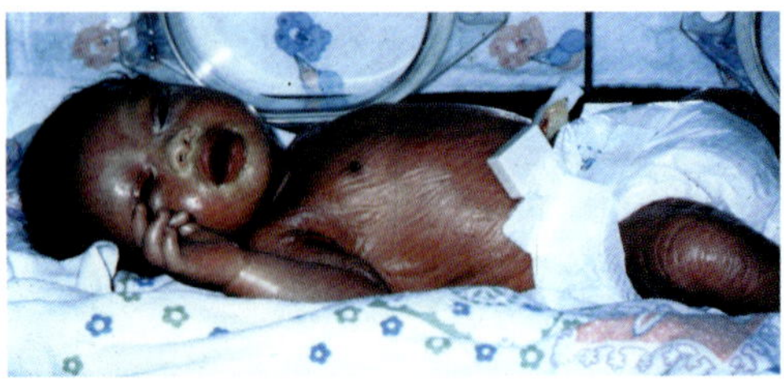

Collodion membrane in a newborn with congenital recessive ichthyosis.

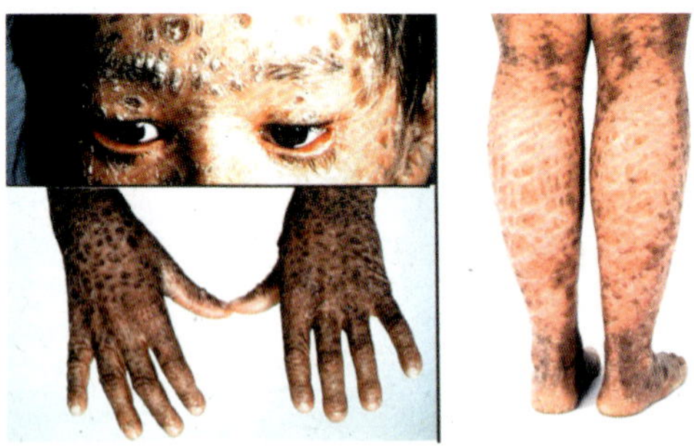

Ectropion (top left), and brown plate-like scale in classic lamellar ichthyosis.

Age of onset

Congenital

Epidemiology 1:200,000 in the US population; 1:91,000 in Norway

Inheritance Autosomal recessive

Chromosomal location 14q11; 2q33-35

Gene TGM1, on 14q11, codes for transglutaminase-1, an enzyme responsible for cross-linking proteins in the formation of the cornified cell envelope. The gene has 15 exons in 14 kb. There is evidence of a second locus for lamellar ichthyosis on chromosome 2, found only in a small group of families from Northern Africa, but no gene has been identified. A few families of Mediterranean origin have been reported where linkage to either chromosome 3 or 19 appears likely.

Mutational spectrum Missense mutations, splice-site mutations and deletions occur throughout the gene.

Effect of mutation Mutations lead to loss of transglutaminase-1 activity which is hypothesized to interfere with normal protein cross-linking and result in production of abnormal cell envelopes in the stratum corneum of the epidermis.

Diagnosis Direct sequence analysis of genomic DNA or analysis of cDNA prepared from a fresh skin biopsy

Counselling issues Few patients, if any, with the strikingly erythrodermic type of congenital recessive ichthyosis have been shown to have mutations in TGM1. However, patients with mild features of lamellar ichthyosis often do. The recurrence risk to siblings of affected children is 25%. Parents of affected children may be consanguineous.

Steroid Sulfatase Deficiency

AKA X-linked ichthyosis

MIM 308100

Clinical features Dark, adherent scale, especially affecting the flexural areas of the body. Asymptomatic corneal opacities. Cryptorchidism, increased risk of testicular cancer.

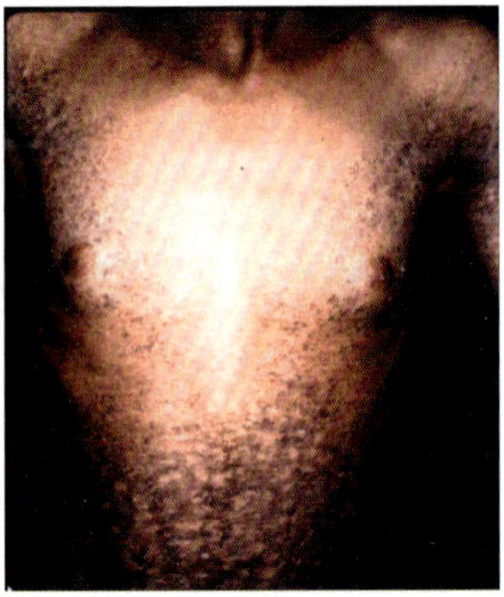

Dark scale, especially affecting the flexures, in steroid sulfatase deficiency.

Age of onset May present at birth with slow progression of labour in the mother and undescended testicles in the affected boy. Ichthyosis is usually evident by six months of age.

Epidemiology Affects 1:2000-6000 males

Inheritance X-linked recessive

Chromosomal location Xp22.32

Gene

STS (previously known as ARSC1), coding for the enzyme steroid sulfatase, a member of the arylsulfatase family. The 146 kb gene codes for a cDNA 2.4 kilobases long.

Mutational spectrum

The majority of mutations (85%) are large deletions of the STS gene. Six patients have been reported who have single base changes, leading to amino acid substitutions in five and premature chain termination in one, all of which are in a 105-amino acid region near the C-terminus of the protein.

Effect of mutation

Lack of activity of the enzyme steroid sulfatase leading to accumulation of undegraded cholesterol sulfate, which is suggested to be responsible for scale-formation in steroid sulfatase deficiency.

Diagnosis

Low oestriol levels in urine/plasma of the mother, due to deficiency of placental steroid sulfatase, indicates an affected foetus. An elevated plasma cholesterol sulfate level (>2000) is diagnostic of an affected male. Direct DNA diagnosis can be made by Southern analysis for the deletions, or by polymerase chain reaction (PCR)-amplification of the STS gene and flanking sequences. Complementary DNA sequence analysis would be required to identify single base substitutions. A method using PCR followed by high performance liquid chromatography (HPLC) and quantification of the PCR products has also been described.

Counselling issues

Family history will often show affected males on maternal side of pedigree (e.g. maternal uncles, nephews, grandfather). Transmission from male to male is not seen. Carrier females may have corneal opacities or mild skin involvement. Contiguous gene syndromes, where the STS gene and another neighbouring gene(s) are deleted, have been characterized many times. Specifically, the association of Kallman syndrome (MIM 147950; characterized by hypogonadotropic hypogonadism and an/hyposmia) with X-linked ichthyosis has been shown to be due to deletions of both the STS and Kallman genes together.

Erythrokeratodermia Variabilis

AKA EKV; Mendes de Costa; Giroux-Barbeau; erythrokeratodermia figurata variabilis; keratosis rubra figurata

MIM 133200

Clinical features Transient erythematous patches that remain for minutes to hours or longer, and hyperkeratosis that can be either generalized, or localized and fixed, with sharply demarcated edges. Palmar-plantar keratoderma is a variable feature. Giroux-Barbeau type is associated with ataxia, usually evident in middle age.

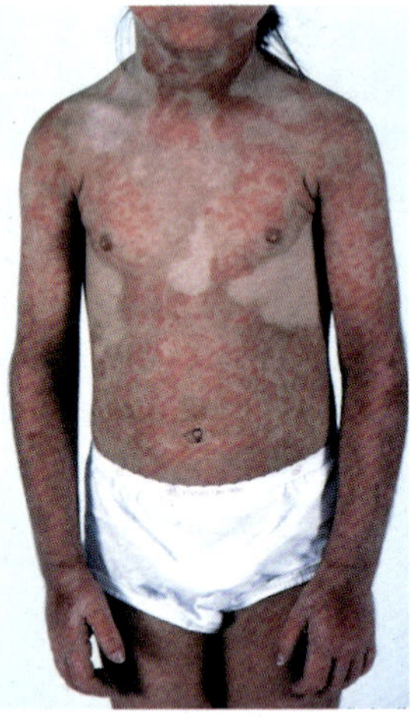

Erythematous patches and hyperkeratosis in erythrokeratodermia variabilis.

Age of onset Infancy; in some patients the erythematous component becomes less prominent with age.

Epidemiology Rare

Inheritance Autosomal dominant

Chromosomal location 1p35.1

Gene GJB3, coding for connexin31, the gap junction protein β-3. The gene has two exons.

Mutational spectrum Single base substitutions identified in many patients with the diagnosis

Effect of mutation Connexins are a multi-gene family of gap-junction proteins responsible for communicating signals between cells. Presumably, the mutated connexin proteins fail to form gap junctions, or form junctions with abnormal function.

Diagnosis Direct sequence analysis of genomic DNA

Counselling issues Although the disease appears to be highly penetrant, some mutation carriers can have extremely mild symptoms and believe themselves to be unaffected. Sporadic or new mutation cases require thorough examination of reportedly unaffected parents, if possible.

Darier Disease

AKA Darier-White disease; keratosis follicularis

MIM 124200

Clinical features Hyperkeratotic, greasy papules that coalesce into plaques in a seborrhoeic distribution, often becoming infected and malodorous. Alternating longitudinal red/white subungual streaks in nails and characteristic v-shaped notching at free edge of nail. Cobblestone papules on oral mucosa. One variant of Darier disease includes haemorrhagic macules and bullae on the palms and soles.

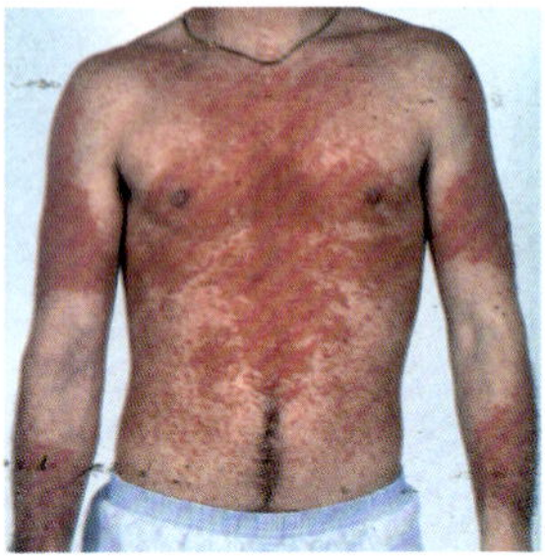

Hyperkeratotic plaques on chest and arms in Darier disease in a young man.

Age of onset Nail changes can often be observed in childhood. Skin changes occur around the age of puberty.

Epidemiology 1:35,000-55,000

Inheritance Autosomal dominant

Chromosomal location 12q24.1

Gene ATP2A2, coding for sarco/endoplasmic reticulum (SER) Ca^{2+}-ATPase isoform 2. The gene has 21 exons.

Mutational spectrum

More than 50% of the mutations lead to premature termination of protein translation, supporting the hypothesis that haplo-insufficiency is responsible for many cases of Darier disease. The remainder of the mutations are missense mutations that occur throughout the gene. One specific missense mutation, $Asn^{767}Ser$, may be associated with the haemorrhagic variant of the disease. Most families have private mutations, i.e. a mutation that has been found only in one family and never observed otherwise.

Effect of mutation

Haplo-insufficiency leading to loss of function of the SER calcium pump is thought to result in abnormal Ca^{2+} signalling in keratinocytes and interference in cell-cell adhesion.

Diagnosis

Histological analyis shows acantholysis, dyskeratosis and corp ronds cells. Molecular diagnosis can be accomplished by sequence analysis of genomic DNA.

Counselling issues

An increased frequency of psychiatric disorders, including depression, has been reported in affected individuals. Anecdotal evidence strongly suggests that the frequency of suicide is also increased. Treatment with lithium (for bipolar disease) can severely exacerbate the skin lesions in these patients.

Hailey-Hailey Disease

AKA Benign familial pemphigus

MIM 169600

Clinical features Skin lesions may begin with transient blistering, progressing to erythematous, scaling plaques, with crusted erosions and fissures. Intertriginous and flexural areas are primarily affected. Lesions are exacerbated by trauma, including heat, sweat and friction. Rarely, faint longitudinal white fingernail lines can be seen.

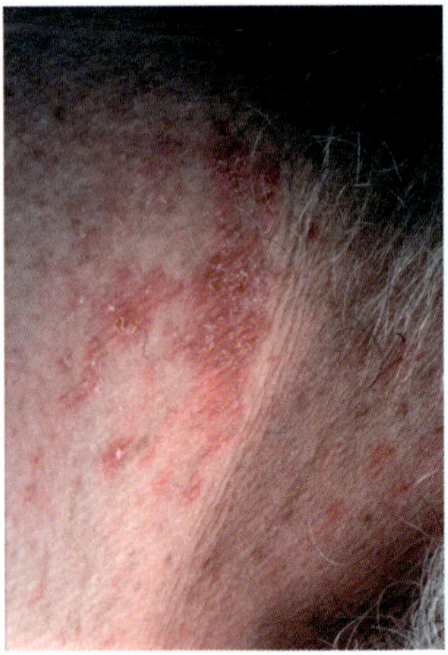

Cluster of erythematous and scaling lesions in the axilla in Hailey-Hailey disease.

Age of onset After puberty, with peak onset between the second and fourth decade

Epidemiology Rare

Inheritance Autosomal dominant

Chromosomal location 3q21-q24

Gene

ATP2C1, a gene coding for an ATP powered calcium pump, containing 27 exons

Mutational spectrum

Frameshift mutations resulting in premature truncation of protein product in more than half of cases. Other mutations include missense, splice-site and nonsense mutations. Two unrelated families have been reported with the same ^{2374}delTTTG mutation.

Effect of mutation

Haplo-insufficiency is the likely cause of clinical symptoms, as supported by the high frequency of predicted protein truncations among the mutations reported. Disease manifestations may be caused by abnormal levels of cytoplasmic or Golgi Ca^{2+} levels.

Diagnosis

Histological features include acantholysis of supra-basal keratinocytes. Single strand conformation polymorphisms (SSCP) or conformation-sensitive gel electrophoresis (CSGE) of PCR-amplified exons, followed by genomic DNA sequence analysis.

Counselling issues

Hailey-Hailey disease is a disorder distinct from Darier disease, although the two share similar histology and both are caused by mutations in genes encoding calcium pumps. The mutations, however, are in different genes on different chromosomes.

Trichothiodystrophy

AKA

PIBIDS; IBIDS; BIDS; Tay syndrome

MIM

278730; 601675

Clinical features

The term trichothiodystrophy means "sulfur-deficient hair". Trichothiodystrophy is actually a group of disorders, from a clinical perspective. Patients may have P = photosensitivity; I1 = ichthyosis; B = brittle hair; I2 = infertility; D = developmental delay; S = short stature. The acronyms above reflect the different constellations of these features seen in individual patients.

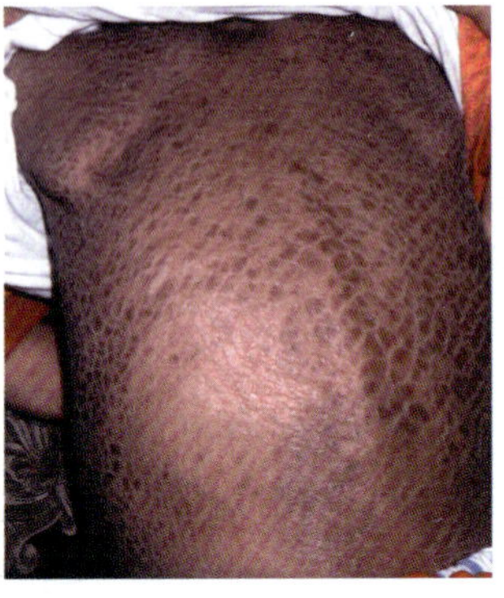

Brown, adherent scale on the back in trichothiodystrophy.

Age of onset

Patients will occasionally present with a collodion membrane at birth; otherwise, the ichthyosis presents neonatally and the sun-sensitivity in infancy.

Epidemiology

Rare, but has been described in all major races

Inheritance

Autosomal recessive

Chromosomal location

19q13 (ERCC2); 2q21 (ERCC3)

Gene

Patients with trichothiodystrophy have mutations in either ERCC2 (more) or ERCC3 (fewer). ERCC2 is the same gene in which mutations are found in xeroderma pigmentosum complementation group D, while ERCC3 mutations are also described in xeroderma pigmentosum complementation group B patients. There is a third group of trichothiodystrophy patients in which the involved gene has not yet been identified.

Mutational spectrum

The site of the mutation in ERCC2 correlates with the clinical phenotype — R^{683} mutations cause xeroderma pigmentosum, while $R^{112}H$, $R^{722}W$ and changes at R^{658} are associated with trichothiodystrophy.

Effect of mutation

ERCC2 and ERCC3 mutations lead to defects in repair of UV-induced DNA damage

Diagnosis

Examination of hair shafts under polarized light reveals a typical tiger tail pattern of alternating light and dark bands. Studies from cultured fibroblasts can identify defective DNA repair. Confirmation of diagnosis using DNA-based methods (sequence analysis of genomic or cDNA) can be performed.

Counselling issues

Despite the overlap with xeroderma pigmentosum and the defective UV-induced DNA repair, risk is very low for development of skin cancer in trichothiodystrophy. Neurological disease in trichothiodystrophy can resemble that seen in Cockayne syndrome (see page 184).

Refsum Disease

AKA	Phytanic acid oxidase deficiency; heredopathica atactica polyneuritiformis
MIM	266500
Clinical features	Retinitis pigmentosa. Progressive polyneuropathy. Cerebellar signs. Nerve deafness. Ichthyosis vulgaris-like skin changes. Anosmia. Multiple epiphyseal dysplasia.
Age of onset	Scaling lesions in childhood or adolescence with retinitis pigmentosa presenting in the second decade of life
Epidemiology	Rare
Inheritance	Autosomal recessive
Chromosomal location	10pter-p11.2
Gene	PAHX, PHYH; coding for phytanoyl-CoA hydroxylase. The open reading frame codes for a 41.2 kDa protein of 338 amino acids.
Mutational spectrum	Deletions and point mutations
Effect of mutation	Inability to metabolise phytanic acid; specifically a defect in the α-oxidation of phytanic acid.
Diagnosis	Increased serum levels of phytanic acid. Mutation analysis of genomic or cDNA may soon become practical to predict recurrence in future pregnancies or identify carriers.
Counselling issues	Restriction of dietary phytanic acid (especially dairy products and chlorophyll-containing foods) leads to improvement in the clinical

symptoms. Plasmapheresis to remove phytanic acid can also help prevent progression of disease.

Epidermolytic Palmoplantar Keratoderma

AKA	Vorner disease
MIM	144200
Clinical features	Yellowish palmar and plantar hyperkeratosis. Patients may have blistering of affected areas, especially with trauma such as friction. The blistering often appears to improve with age.

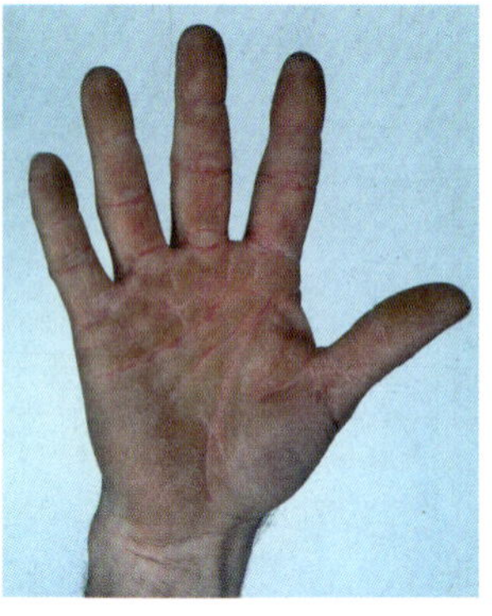

Palm in epidermolytic palmar-plantar keratoderma.

Age of onset	At birth or in the neonatal period. The palm and sole skin often appears thicker and whitish at this time. A single transverse palmar crease, representative of restricted hand movement during foetal life due to the hyperkeratosis, is common.
Epidemiology	May be more frequent in Northern Europeans than other ethnic groups
Inheritance	Autosomal dominant
Chromosomal location	17q12-q21

Gene

KRT9, coding for keratin 9, a type II neutral/basic epidermal keratin. The gene contains 8 exons.

Mutational spectrum

Single base substitutions leading to amino acid changes in the highly conserved coil 1A of the rod domain of the keratin protein. $Arg^{162}Trp$ has been seen in several families.

Effect of mutation

Mutations are expected to interfere with the assembly of keratin proteins into intermediate filaments in the keratinocytes. Keratins are usually expressed in pairs, and mutation of either one of a pair generally leads to the same or very similar clinical expression. However, the expression partner of keratin 9 has not yet been identified.

Diagnosis

Histological examination of affected skin shows epidermolysis of supra-basal keratinocytes. Direct sequence analysis of genomic DNA identifies disease-associated point mutations in KRT9.

Counselling issues

There are many types of palmoplantar keratoderma. The histological evidence of epidermolysis and restriction of the clinical phenotype to the palms and soles, but in a generalized rather than punctate or striate distribution, helps identify the Vorner subtype.

Non-epidermolytic Palmoplantar Keratoderma

AKA Unna-Thost disease

MIM 600962

Clinical features Diffuse hyperkeratosis of palms and soles, often with a distinct erythematous border at the volar/dorsal margin.

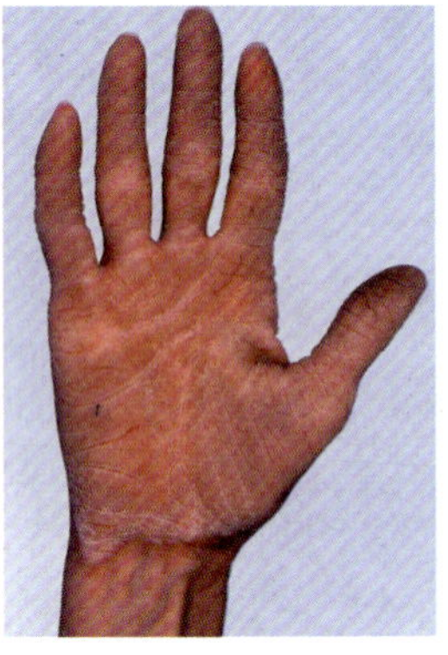

Palm in non-epidermolytic palmar-plantar keratoderma.

Age of onset By one year of age

Inheritance Autosomal dominant

Chromosomal location 12q11-q13; 17q12-q21

Genes Mutations in either KRT1, coding for keratin 1 (chromosome 12), or KRT16, coding for keratin 16 (chromosome 17), have been described.

Mutational spectrum In KRT1, a mutation affecting the variable region (V1 domain) of the protein, $Lys^{73}Ile$, has been described in a large kindred. Some families have also shown linkage to the type II (neutral/basic) keratin gene cluster on chromosome 12, but the specific keratin gene involved has not been identified. Other families have been found to have mutations in KRT16, a type I keratin gene located on chromosome 17. The specific mutations in KRT16 so far described result in the following amino acid substitutions: $Arg^{10}Cys$ and $Asn^{8}Ser$.

Effect of mutation

The $Lys^{73}Ile$ protein change resulting from the KRT1 mutation is hypothesized to interfere with keratin interactions with intermediate filament associated proteins. The KRT16 mutations affect the helix initiation motif of the 1A domain of the keratin 16 protein, and probably interfere with the keratin protein's ability to form filaments.

Diagnosis

No evidence of epidermolysis will be seen on light microscopy, in contrast to Vorner syndrome. In large families, linkage analysis may identify the suspect keratin. KRT1 and KRT16 mutation analysis can then be achieved by sequencing genomic DNA.

Counselling issues

There are forms of non-epidermolytic palmoplantar hyperkeratosis that map to chromosome 17q23-qter rather than to the keratin cluster at 17q12-q21. These families usually have a focal, rather than diffuse, distribution of their keratoderma. In many of these families, the keratoderma is associated with oesophageal cancer, and the disorder is designated tylosis with oesophageal cancer (MIM 148500). The gene has not yet been identified. A family history should be obtained from any patient with palmoplantar keratoderma to assess the presence of gastrointestinal cancer, especially oesophageal.

Hereditary Palmoplantar Keratoderma Striata

AKA

Brunauer-Fuhs-Siemens palmoplantar keratoderma; keratosis palmoplantaris striata

MIM

148700

Clinical features

Linear pattern of hyperkeratotic streaks on palms and flexor surface of fingers with islands of thickening on soles, and no tendency to blister.

Age of onset

First to second decade

Inheritance

Autosomal dominant

Chromosomal location

18q12.1-q12.2; 6p2

Gene

The clinical features have been shown to map to either of two chromosomal locations, in different families. Mutations in genes coding for the components of the desmosome have been identified: DSG1, coding for desmoglein 1, on chromosome 18; and DSP, coding for desmoplakin, on chromosome 6. Desmosomes are specialized structures in the plasma membrane that act as a junction between epithelial cells. Desmoglein I is a member of the cadherin cell adhesion molecule family. Desmoplakin is located at the intercellular side of the desmosome and is one of several plaken proteins that mediate interaction of the cytoskeleton with desmosomes.

Mutational spectrum

One mutation in a single family has been described to date in DSP; a C to T transition in exon 4 leading to Gln^{331}Ter and premature truncation of the desmoplakin protein. Similarly, a single mutation in DSG1 has been described; a splice-acceptor site mutation resulting in in-frame deletion of exon 3.

Effect of mutation

Interference with cadherin function and resultant abnormality of the desmosome, probably due to haplo-insufficiency of the affected protein.

Diagnosis

Linkage studies followed by sequence analysis of cDNA

Counselling issues

Linkage studies in affected families will determine which gene to sequence for mutation identification.

Vohwinkel Syndrome

AKA	Hereditary palmoplantar keratoderma Vohwinkel; keratodermia hereditaria mutilans
MIM	124500
Clinical features	Diffuse honeycomb hyperkeratosis of palms and soles with typical starfish keratoses on dorsum of hands and feet. Pseudo-ainhum (constricting bands) sometimes leading to autoamputation of digits. Moderate degree of hearing loss to deafness.
Age of onset	Hyperkeratosis in neonatal period; constricting bands develop in early childhood. The deafness can be congenital.
Epidemiology	Reported in many European ethnic groups
Inheritance	Autosomal dominant
Chromosomal location	13q11-q12
Gene	GJB2, coding for connexin 26 (Cx26), a β-2 gap-junction protein. The gene has two exons, one of which encodes the 26 kDa protein.
Mutational spectrum	$Asp^{66}His$ has been found in British, Spanish and Italian Vohwinkel pedigrees.
Effect of mutation	Connexins are a multi-gene family of proteins that form gap-junctions between cells. Gap junctions allow selective ion exchange and communicate signals between cells. Presumably, the mutated connexin proteins form abnormal junctions, or junctions with abnormal function.

Diagnosis

Direct sequence analysis of genomic DNA

Counselling issues

There are other autosomal dominant palmoplantar keratodermas that are associated with congenital deafness. GJB2 mutations have also been identified in families who do not have the skin findings characteristic of Vohwinkel syndrome, including the $R^{75}W$ and $M^{34}T$ mutations.

Loricrin Keratoderma

AKA Variant form of Vohwinkel syndrome

MIM 604117

Clinical features Palmar and plantar honeycomb hyperkeratosis with pseudo-ainhum. Diffuse generalized ichthyosis. No hearing loss (in contrast to true Vohwinkel syndrome, see page 28).

Age of onset By 18 months.

Epidemiology Original family emigrated to the United States from the United Kingdom in the mid 1700s

Chromosomal location 1q21

Gene LOR, coding for loricrin. The LOR gene is 2.5 kb long, has a single intron in the 5′-untranslated portion of the gene, and no introns interrupting the coding sequence. LOR is one member of the epidermal differentiation complex, which is a cluster of genes on 1q important in epidermal differentiation. Loricrin is one of the proteins crosslinked by transglutaminase to form the cell envelope of corneocytes.

Mutational spectrum Single base insertions that cause a frameshift and delayed termination of protein translation, i.e. a longer than normal protein product

Effect of mutation It is hypothesized that this mutation leads to a gain of function (a new function due to the different sequence and structure) of the loricrin protein.

Diagnosis Direct sequence analysis of genomic DNA

Counselling issues A LOR mutation has also been described in a single family with progressive symmetric erythrokeratoderma (PSEK). Patients shared many clinical features with the family originally described with loricrin keratoderma.

Mal de Meleda

AKA	Keratosis palmoplantaris transgradiens of Siemens; Mal de Mljet
MIM	248300
Clinical features	Diffuse palmar and plantar hyperkeratosis with restricted extension of digits. Hyperhidrosis. Hyperkeratosis also seen on extensor surfaces of joints and axillae. Transgradiens involvement. Various morphological and functional cardiac anomalies. Perioral erythema.
Age of onset	Infancy
Epidemiology	Initially described among inhabitants of the island of Meleda in Palmatia, Yugoslavia (Adriatic Sea), but since reported in other ethnic groups from Europe, particularly Greece.
Inheritance	Autosomal recessive
Chromosomal location	8qter
Gene	Unknown. Linkage to the marker D8S1751. The candidate region has been narrowed to about 3 million basepairs of DNA, distal to marker D8S1727.
Mutational spectrum	Unknown
Diagnosis	Still a clinical diagnosis, although linkage analysis in informative families may be confirmative
Counselling issues	Knowledge of the ethnic origin of affected individuals can help in the differential diagnosis.

Papillon-Lefevre

AKA	Keratosis palmoplantaris with periodontopathia
MIM	245000
Clinical features	Palmar plantar hyperkeratosis. Severe early-onset periodontitis. Hypotrichosis. Hypodontia. Fragile nails.
Age of onset	Palmoplantar hyperkeratosis develops in the first 3 years of life. Patients are usually ascertained by a dentist following treatment for periodontal disease.
Epidemiology	Parental consanguinity is a frequent finding. The disease has been described in diverse ethnic populations, including Arab, Turk, German and Ethiopian.
Inheritance	Autosomal recessive
Chromosomal location	11q14.1-q14.3
Gene	CTSC, encoding the lysosomal protease cathepsin C. The CTSC message is highly expressed in polymorphonuclear leukocytes, alveolar macrophages and their precursor cells. The CTSC gene has 7 exons.
Mutational spectrum	From a series of 8 families, mostly missense and nonsense mutations were identified. One mutation altering a splice site was also observed.
Effect of mutation	Total loss of cathepsin C activity, possibly leading to reduced host response to bacteria in dental plaque and other sites.

Diagnosis Direct sequence analysis of genomic DNA

Counselling issues Haim Munk syndrome is in the differential diagnosis, with palmoplantar keratoderma, periodontal disease, and leukocyte adhesion deficiency. The skin lesions are similar to those seen in Mal de Meleda (see page 32). Obligate carriers of a CTSC mutation have been shown to have reduced activity of cathepsin C in a functional assay.

Richner-Hanhart Syndrome

AKA	Tyrosine transaminase deficiency; tyrosinaemia type II
MIM	276600
Clinical features	Blisters on palms, soles and fingertips progressing to painful punctate keratoses. Corneal ulcers. Mental retardation in some.
Age of onset	Early childhood to late teens
Epidemiology	Many of the reported cases are of Italian ancestry
Inheritance	Autosomal recessive
Chromosomal location	16q22.1-q22.3
Gene	TAT, coding for the enzyme tyrosine amino transferase. The gene has 12 exons and extends over 10.9 kb.
Mutational spectrum	Point mutations, most of which result in early stop codons
Effect of mutation	Deficiency of the hepatic enzyme amino transferase, probably with accumulation of tyrosine crystals in keratinocytes (as suggested by electron microscopic studies).
Diagnosis	Sequence analysis of genomic DNA. Prenatal diagnosis by molecular methods in at-risk pregnancies.
Counselling issues	Even within families, the clinical features can be quite variable.

2. Genodermatoses with Malignant Potential

Xeroderma Pigmentosum

AKA XPA; XPB; XPC; XPD; XPE; XPF; XPG; XPVariant

MIM 278700-278800

Clinical features Skin photosensitivity with early onset of poikilodermatous changes including hypo- and hyper pigmentation, freckles, lentigines, skin atrophy and multiple skin cancers (basal cell, squamous cell and melanoma). Photophobia. Keratitis. Conjunctivitis. Ectropion. Mental deterioration. Ataxia. Spasticity. Neurological findings especially in XPA.

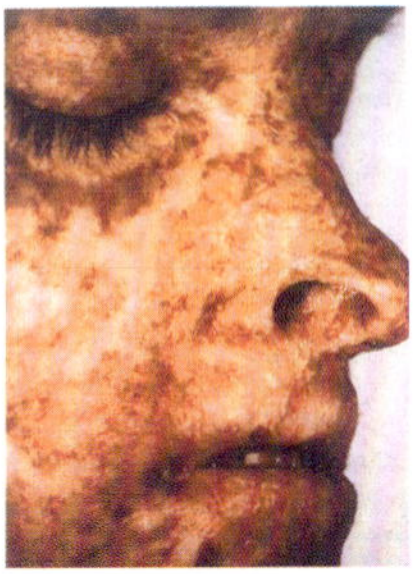

16 year old showing skin changes of xeroderma pigmentosum. Photo courtesy of K.H. Kraemer, M.D.

Age of onset Skin changes in early childhood; neurological and ophthalmologic changes are progressive over time.

Epidemiology Although rare, XP has been described in populations worldwide. It is not uncommon for parents to be consanguineous. XPA is most common, and accounts for nearly all Japanese patients. It is also the most common type of XP in Egypt.

Inheritance Autosomal recessive

Chromosomal location XP genes have been localized to 9q22.3 (XPA), 2q21

(XPB/ERCC3), 3p25 (XPC), 19q13.2 (XPD/ERCC2), 11p12 (XPE/DDB2), 16p13.3 (XPF/ERCC4) and 13q13 (XPG/ERCC5).

Genes

XPA (type A), XPB/ERCC3 (type B), XPC (type C), XPD/ERCC2 (type D), XPE/DDB2 (type E), XPF/ERCC4 (type F) and XPG/ERCC5 (type G). XPVariant is caused by mutations in POLH (chromosome location unknown) which codes for DNA polymerase eta.

Mutational spectrum

Mutations of each of the XP-associated genes show wide variation, with frequent small deletions, missense and nonsense mutations, and mutations affecting splice sites. XPC also has large deletions. $Arg^{788}Trp$ in ERCC4 has been seen many times. POLH has been found to have deletions and nonsense mutations resulting in truncated proteins.

Effect of mutation

Mutations in the genes associated with XP impair the ability of cells to repair UV-induced DNA damage.

Diagnosis

Skin fibroblasts from XP patients show defective DNA repair of UV-induced photoproducts. Complementation studies can identify the specific complementation group. Direct mutation analysis of the specific XP gene associated with that complementation group can often be performed and the results used to identify heterozygous carriers in a family, as well as for pre-natal diagnosis in at-risk pregnancies.

Counselling issues

XP with severe neurological abnormalities and dwarfism is also called De Sanctis Cacchione syndrome. Mutations in XPB, XPD and XPG have been found in patients who have both XP and Cockayne syndrome (see page 184). It is unclear what the relationship is between Cockayne syndrome without XP and the type that occurs in the context of XP. Mutations in XPB and XPD are also associated with trichothiodystrophy (see page 18).

Naevoid Basal Cell Carcinoma Syndrome

AKA

Gorlin syndrome; basal cell naevus syndrome; Gorlin-Goltz syndrome

MIM

109400

Clinical features

Classic triad of multiple basal cell carcinomas developing at a young age. Odontogenic keratocysts. Pits of the palms and soles. Multiple skeletal anomalies including ectopic calcification, especially of the falx cerebri and rib and spine malformations. Coarse facial features with prominent mandible and frontal and biparietal bossing (prominence).

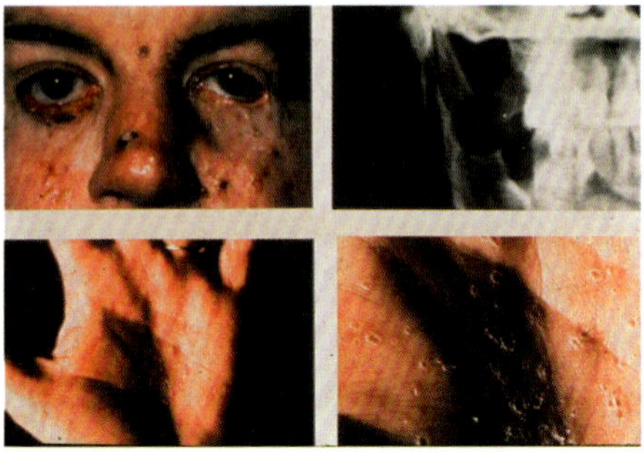

Gorlin syndrome. Top left, multiple basal cell carcinomas. Top right, radiograph showing large jaw cyst in the mandible. Bottom left, palmar pits. Bottom right, palmar pits become more prominent after soaking the hand in warm water.

Age of onset

Skin cancers usually develop in late teens but can be seen in early childhood; jaw cysts usually develop around puberty.

Epidemiology

All races and ethnicities can be affected, although dark-skinned individuals have fewer skin cancers. Approximately 1/3 of cases result from a new dominant mutation.

Inheritance

Autosomal dominant

Chromosomal location

9q22.3

Gene

PTCH, the human homologue of Drosophila *patched*. The patched protein is the cell surface receptor for the *hedgehog* protein and is involved in the *hedgehog* signalling pathway. The PTCH gene has 22 exons.

Mutation spectrum

Approximately 80% of PTCH mutations result in premature truncation of the patched protein. Mutations occur throughout the gene.

Effect of mutation

Absence of sufficient patched protein to bind to hedgehog protein in the cell membrane is hypothesized to release the smoothened protein from its normally suppressed state. Smoothened is then free to initiate a signalling cascade involving several proteins important in cell growth and differentiation. The PTCH gene is considered to be a tumour suppressor gene, which follows Knudson's Two-Hit hypothesis. The first hit is the inherited mutation in PTCH. This is thought to lead to haplo-insufficiency of patched protein and resultant developmental defects associated with the syndrome. The second hit occurs when the normal PTCH gene is mutated in a somatic cell, leading to absence or greatly reduced amounts of normal patched protein. This is thought to result in cutaneous (and any other) malignancies associated with the syndrome.

Diagnosis

Mutation detection involves screening of the entire PTCH gene for mutations using either SSCP, di-deoxyfingerprinting (ddF) or direct sequence analysis of genomic DNA.

Counselling issues

Approximately 5% of infants with Gorlin syndrome develop medulloblastoma. Radiation treatment for the medulloblastoma can result in a crop of basal cell carcinomas in the radiation port. One-third of females with Gorlin syndrome have ovarian fibromas which, if left untreated, can impair fertility. The fibromas have a slight risk of degenerating into ovarian fibrosarcoma.

Cowden Syndrome

AKA Multiple hamartoma syndrome

MIM 158350

Clinical features Hamartomas of the skin, mucous membranes, breast and thyroid. Facial tricholemmomas. Papillomas of the skin. Cobble-stoning of oral mucosal. Keratoses of palms and soles. Associated anomalies of multiple organ systems include colonic polyposis, skeletal findings (scoliosis, pectus excavatum) and menstrual irregularities.

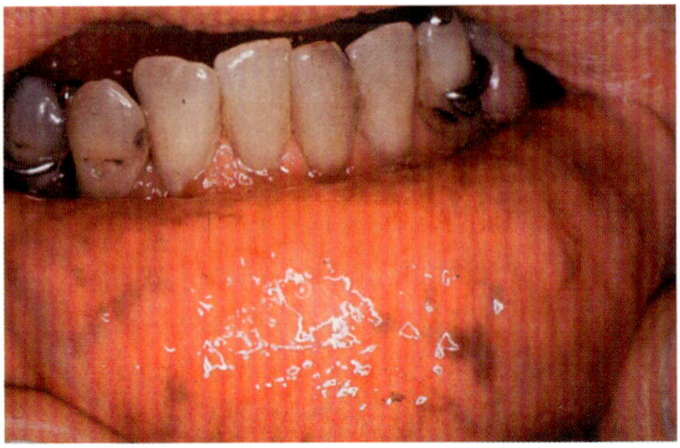

Multiple mucosal papules on the lower lip in Cowden syndrome. Photo courtesy of J.R. Toro, MD.

Age of onset Skin findings usually evident by 20 years of age

Epidemiology One in 200,000-250,000, as estimated from the Dutch population

Inheritance Autosomal dominant

Chromosomal location 10q23.3

Gene PTEN, deriving its name from the observation of *p*hosphatase and *ten*sin homologue deleted on chromosome 10. PTEN has 9 exons and codes for a 403 amino acid protein.

Mutational spectrum

Many missense and nonsense mutations dispersed throughout the gene. There is a possible cluster of mutations reported in exon 5. Mutations are not identified in some patients with Cowden syndrome even when the extended family shows linkage to the chromosome 10q23.3 region, implying that there are portions of the gene that have not yet been identified.

Effect of mutation

PTEN appears to function as a tumour suppressor gene, and loss of heterozygosity at chromosome 10q23 is seen in a variety of tumour types.

Diagnosis

Direct sequencing of genomic DNA

Counselling issues

There is an increased risk of malignancy in patients with Cowden syndrome, especially gynaecological malignancies, and breast, thyroid, bladder and renal cancers. These patients require regular screening for associated malignancies and appropriate surveillance. It has been proposed that Bannayan-Riley-Ruvalcaba syndrome (MIM 153480) is allelic to Cowden syndrome.

Gardner Syndrome

AKA	Familial adenomatous polyposis (FAP) with extra-intestinal tumours
MIM	175100
Clinical features	Epidermoid cysts and fibromas of the skin. Osteomas of skull and mandible. Colon, duodenum and gastric polyps (often numbering in the thousands), that have a high risk of malignant transformation. Desmoid tumours. Congenital hypertrophy of retinal pigment epithelium (CHRPE).
Age of onset	CHRPE is congenital and should be evident in infancy. Skin lesions develop during childhood and puberty. Intestinal polyps develop in second decade.
Epidemiology	Estimates from the Dutch show a frequency of 1:13,500. Penetrance is nearly 100% by age 40. The proportion of Gardner syndrome cases due to new mutations is thought to be approximately 25%.
Inheritance	Autosomal dominant
Chromosomal location	5q21-q22
Gene	APC, a molecule involved in the cell signalling pathway. Among other functions, APC protein is thought to regulate β-catenin levels in normal cells.
Mutational spectrum	There is a mutational cluster region in the central portion of the gene. Mutations mostly result in truncated proteins. Mutations in the 3′- and 5′-ends of the gene are associated with attenuation of the clinical features (later onset, fewer polyps). Approximately 25% of Ashkenazi Jewish patients with colon cancer have a specific APC

mutation, $I^{1307}K$. However, the increased risk of colon cancer associated with this mutation, as judged from population studies of unselected individuals, appears to be only moderate.

Effect of mutation

Mutations in APC are thought to cause symptomatology through a dominant negative effect. Loss of heterozygosity for the APC gene is seen frequently in both Gardner syndrome-associated colonic tumours and sporadic tumours of the colon.

Diagnosis

At-risk persons can be identified by the presence of CHRPE. Linkage analysis can be performed in informative families. Direct cDNA sequence analysis of APC can be performed, using denaturing gradient gel electrophoresis (DGGE) for exons 1-14 and a protein truncation assay for the large exon 15.

Counselling issues

Increased risk of various malignancies including periampullary carcinoma, hepatoblastoma, bile duct, adrenal and thyroid carcinoma, and osteosarcoma. Presence of CHRPE can identify those individuals in the family who will benefit from intensive surveillance for Gardner syndrome-associated tumours.

Fanconi Anaemia

AKA	Fanconi pancytopaenia
MIM	227650 (Group A); 227660 (Group B); 227645 (Group C); 227646 (Group D); 600901 (Group E); 603467 (Group F); 602956 (Group G); 603468 (Group H), based on complementation groups
Clinical features	Pigmentary changes (diffuse or patchy, hyper- or hypo-pigmentation, café-au-lait spots and freckling). Bruisability. Anaemic pallor. Radial aplasia with aplastic, hypoplastic, deformed or duplicated thumb. Bone marrow failure. Growth retardation. Microcephaly and mental retardation (about 25%). Eye, ear, heart and genitourinary malformations.
Cytogenetics	High frequency of spontaneous chromosome and chromatid breaks. Rearrangements, especially formation of quadriradials observed in cultured cells, as well as those exposed to DNA cross-linking agents such as diepoxybutane and mitomycin C.
Age of onset	Congenital
Epidemiology	Group A is the most common complementation group among North American patients and Germans, representing 2/3 of cases. The second most common type in these patients was Group C, which also accounts for the majority of patients in the Netherlands. Incidence of Fanconi anaemia estimated in white, Afrikaans-speaking South Africans is 1:22,000 with the heterozygote frequency 1:77. In this population there appears to be a founder effect.

Chromosomal location

Fanconi anaemia loci have been identified on 16q24.3 (Group A); 9q22.3 (Group C); 3p26-p22 (Group D); 6p22-p21 (Group E); and 9p13 (Group G).

Genes

The FAA gene on 16q24.3 (which codes for a polypeptide of 1455 amino acids) is responsible for Group A Fanconi anaemia, and the FAC gene (which codes for a 557 amino acid protein, and contains 14 exons in 1.6kb) is responsible for Group C Fanconi anaemia. However, the genes responsible for the other complementation groups have yet to be identified. Mutations in XRCC9, which has no similarity to any other known protein, have been identified in Fanconi anaemia Group G.

Mutation spectrum

In FAA, a high frequency of intragenic deletions is found which remove up to 31 exons of the gene. Two small deletions, $^{1115\text{-}1118}$del and $^{3788\text{-}3790}$del, accounted for 2% and 5% of the FAA alleles in one large study. FAC mutations include missense and nonsense changes, as well as small deletions and insertions. Two mutations in XRCC9 have been identified: Glu^{105}Ter and a splice acceptor mutation.

Effect of mutation

It is hypothesized that the FAA gene is hypermutable. Many of the large deletions in FAA delete Alu repeats and it is suggested that Alu-mediated recombination may be a mechanism for development of anaemia in the disease. The FAC gene protein localizes primarily to the cytoplasm of the cell and is therefore thought to have only an indirect role in regulating DNA repair. It has been shown that the FAA and FAC proteins bind each other and form a complex, suggesting the inter-relatedness of these genes in a DNA repair pathway.

Diagnosis

SSCP screening of FAA cDNA

Counselling issues

Leukaemia is a fatal complication of Fanconi anaemia, with mean age at death occurring before 10 years of age. Leukaemia may also occur in family members who do not have the full-blown features of the disease. There is a suggestion that Blackfan-Diamond hypoplastic anaemia is allelic to Fanconi anaemia.

Bloom Syndrome

MIM

210900

Clinical features

Sun-sensitive skin with facial erythema, in a butterfly distribution across the nose and cheeks. Telangiectasia. Atrophy with hypo- and hyper-pigmentary changes. Growth failure of pre-natal onset, and resultant short stature. Thin face with malar hypoplasia. Severe immunodeficiency and recurrent infections. Pulmonary fibrosis and bronchiectasis. Cardiomyopathy. High risk of malignancy of various organs. Decreased fertility.

Cytogenetics

High rate of sister chromatid exchange observed on metaphase spreads of chromosomes

Age of onset

Infancy

Epidemiology

Rare, but affects members of many ethnic groups. There is a significantly higher frequency in Jewish people, especially those of Ashkenazi background, where a founder effect has caused nearly all affected individuals to have the identical mutation. Parental consanguinity is common in the parents of affected children.

Inheritance

Autosomal recessive

Chromosomal location

15q26.1

Gene

BLM, which codes for a protein that has homology to other members of a family of DNA helicases (proteins that unwind DNA).

Mutational spectrum

Small deletions and insertions, and missense mutations. The mutation in most Ashkenazi Jewish patients is a 6 bp deletion/7 bp insertion at nucleotide 2281 of the BLM cDNA.

Effect of mutation

It is proposed that mutations in the BLM gene cause changes that interfere with the resultant protein's normal interaction with topoisomerases. It has also been observed that altered DNA ligase I activity is a consistent feature of Bloom syndrome cells.

Diagnosis

A simple PCR-based test is available to screen for the Ashkenazi mutation and can be used to identify heterozygous carriers in a family or population.

Counselling issues

Death usually occurs by early adulthood in patients with Bloom syndrome.

Ataxia Telangiectasia

AKA	Louis-Bar syndrome
MIM	208900
Clinical features	Oculocutaneous telangiectasias. Cerebellar ataxia. Immune defects. Increased risk for malignancy.
Cytogenetics	High frequency of chromosome breaks and re-arrangements
Age of onset	Cerebellar ataxia usually presents in early childhood. The telangiectasias develop between the ages of 3 and 5 years, with oculomotor apraxia often preceding the appearance of the conjunctival telangiectasias.
Epidemiology	Incidence is approximately 1 in 11 million births, estimated in the US Caucasian population. The heterozygote frequency has been estimated at 2.8%.
Inheritance	Autosomal recessive
Chromosomal location	11q22.3
Gene	ATM, encoding a large protein kinase with a PI-3 kinase-related domain. The gene is involved in mitogenic signal transduction, meiotic recombination and cell-cycle control, and is activated in cells with damaged DNA. There are 66 exons in the ATM gene, and the transcript is 12 kb long.
Mutational spectrum	There are a wide variety of mutations, with specific ethnic populations often having one or two more frequent mutations. For example, ^{4612}Del165 and ^{7883}Del5 in Japanese and ^{3245}ATC→TGAT in Norwegians.

Effect of mutation

There are at least four different ataxia telangiectasia complementation groups. Three of the groups (A,C,D) comprise 97% of the cases, and each of these maps to 11q22.3. It is possible that specific mutations in ATM account for the different cellular phenotypes (complementation groups). Alternatively, it may be that there is more than one ataxia telangiectasia gene in close proximity on 11q22.3.

Diagnosis

Prenatal diagnosis by linkage analysis has been performed. Screening of cDNA using PCR-SSCP methods is suggested as a first stage approach to mutation identification.

Counselling issues

Patients have an increased sensitivity to ionizing radiation. There is a strong predisposition to malignancy, especially leukaemia, but also to solid tumours including medulloblastoma and glioma. Some studies have suggested that heterozygotes for mutations in ATM have an increased risk for breast cancer (2-5 times higher than the general population).

Rothmund-Thomson Syndrome

AKA	Poikiloderma atrophicans and cataract; hereditary poikiloderma congenitale
MIM	268400
Clinical features	Poikilodermatous skin changes including atrophy, pigmentary changes and telangiectasia. Alopecia. Cataract. Congenital bone defects including metaphyseal chondrodysplasia. Hypogonadism. Hypodontia.
Age of onset	Poikilodermatous changes usually seen within the first year of life
Epidemiology	Approximately 150 cases have been reported in the literature
Inheritance	Autosomal recessive
Chromosomal location	8q24.3
Gene	RECQL4, a DNA helicase (unwinding) gene. The gene is 6.5 kb long, and contains 21 exons.
Mutation spectrum	Only a few mutations have been reported to date, including a 7 bp deletion, a single base substitution resulting in a stop codon, a 2 bp deletion and a single base substitution that alters a splice acceptor site.
Effect of mutation	Mutations are hypothesized to interfere with the helicase function of the protein that unwinds double stranded DNA into single stranded DNA.
Diagnosis	Sequence analysis of genomic DNA

Counselling issues

Patients with Rothmund-Thomson syndrome have an increased risk for developing osteosarcoma, especially of long bones in areas of metaphyseal chrondrodysplasia. Also, there is a questionable increased risk of skin cancer.

Muir-Torre Syndrome

AKA

Muir-Torre syndrome appears to be a variant of Lynch Cancer Family Syndrome Type II (a subset of hereditary non-polyposis colon cancer)

MIM

158320

Clinical features

Sebaceous tumours including adenomas, epitheliomas, carcinomas and basal cell epitheliomas with sebaceous differentiation. Keratoacanthomas. Internal malignancies including colon duodenal, laryngeal and endometrial malignancies.

Age of onset

Adulthood

Epidemiology

Mutations in MSH2 also occur in Lynch Cancer Family Syndrome Type II, and mutations in MLH1 account for many cases of hereditary non-polyposis colon cancer, a fairly common disorder. Muir-Torre syndrome, in which the skin findings are clinically significant, appears to be a rare variant of the other, more common, non-polyposis colon cancer syndromes.

Inheritance

Autosomal dominant

Chromosomal location

2p22-p21; 3p21.3

Genes

MSH2 on chromosome 2 contains 16 exons over 73 kb of genomic DNA. This gene is homologous to MutS, a gene in the DNA mismatch repair system in *Escherichia coli* and *Saccharomyces cerevisiae.* MLH1 on chromosome 3 is related to bacterial and yeast MutL genes, also involved in mismatch repair. MLH1 has 19 exons spanning 100 kb.

Mutational spectrum

MSH2 mutations all result in stop codons, either directly or through frameshifts. MLH1 mutations are also large deletions resulting in truncated proteins.

Effect of mutation

Mutations interfere with the ability of these proteins to repair DNA mismatches that occur during DNA replication.

Diagnosis

MSH2 mutations have been identified using DGGE and direct genomic DNA sequencing. MLH1 mutations can be screened using SSCP of PCR-amplified fragments and genomic DNA sequencing of fragments with abnormal SSCP patterns. Protein truncation tests have also been utilized in mutation detection.

Counselling issues

There are significantly more mutations in MSH2 than in MLH1 in Muir-Torre patients, so genetic screening for mutations should be done with this in mind.

Cutaneous Malignant Melanoma

AKA Hereditary dysplastic naevus syndrome; familial multiple mole and melanoma syndrome

MIM 155600

Clinical features Multiple primary melanomas are not uncommon. Many patients also have multiple clinically abnormal and histologically dysplastic pigmented naevi distributed over both sun-exposed and sun-protected areas of the body. Cutaneous malignant melanoma.

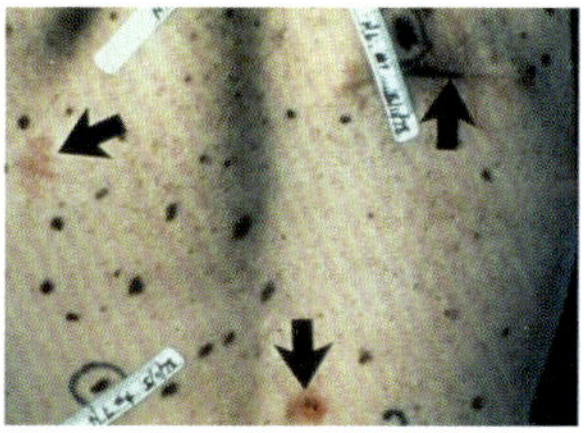

Multiple atypical naevi and malignant melanoma in familial cutaneous malignant melanoma.

Age of onset Melanoma can occur as early as childhood. Abnormal moles are usually observable in late childhood or at the onset of puberty.

Epidemiology More common in fair-skinned, light-eyed people. Sun exposure is an important determinant of risk of melanoma. The presence of dysplastic naevi increases the risk of melanoma independent of whether or not a patient has a mutation in one of the identified risk genes.

Inheritance Autosomal dominant

Chromosomal location 9p21; 1p36; 12q13

Gene CDKN2A (also known as p16 or p16INK4), coding for cyclin-dependent kinase inhibitor-2A on chromosome 9p. The gene has 3 exons. Another locus appears to exist on 1p36 (no gene yet identified) and accounts for a subset of familial melanoma in which the dysplastic naevi are a prominent feature. CDK4, on chromosome 12q, codes for cyclin-dependent kinase 4 and has 8 exons.

Mutational spectrum

In CDKN2A, the gene responsible for most of the mutations in this disease thus far identified, nonsense, missense, deletion and insertion mutations occur. Exon 2 of CDKN2A is a priority site for mutations. For CDK4, mutations have been found in exon 2A which inhibits binding to the p16 protein.

Effect of mutations

CDKN2A is a tumour suppressor gene. Inactivation of the gene causes loss of normal cell-cycle arrest in the late G1 phase. In familial cutaneous malignant melanoma, the first CDKN2A mutation is inherited from a parent, while the second event is mutation or deletion of the homologous copy of the gene in the somatic cell, leading to development of the cutaneous lesion.

Diagnosis

Direct sequence analysis of the CDKN2A gene from genomic DNA. It is suggested that screening of the promoter region may be useful in identifying mutations in patients of Northern European ancestry. Failing identification of mutations in this gene, CDK4 can also be screened.

Counselling issues

The abnormal naevi are thought to be precursor lesions, and some have a high risk of developing into melanoma over time. This fact allows a means for management and prevention, e.g. regular visual examination of the total body surface, biopsy of lesions showing changes and early excision of suspicious lesions. However, melanomas can arise independently of these abnormal naevi. There may also be an increased risk for development of pancreatic cancer in a small subset of families. Mutations in CDKN2 or CDK4 indicate an increased risk of development of melanoma. However, it can not be inferred that an individual with such a mutation will definitely develop the disease. These mutations are considered predisposition alleles and occur only in a subset of families.

Multiple Endocrine Neoplasia Type I

AKA

Wermer syndrome; multiple endocrine adenomatosis

MIM

131100

Clinical features

Peptic ulcer disease. Endocrine abnormalities involving the pituitary and parathyroid glands, and the pancreas. Skin findings in this disorder have only recently been characterized, and consist of multiple facial angiofibromas, collagenomas and lipomas, confetti-like hypopigmented macules and gingival papules.

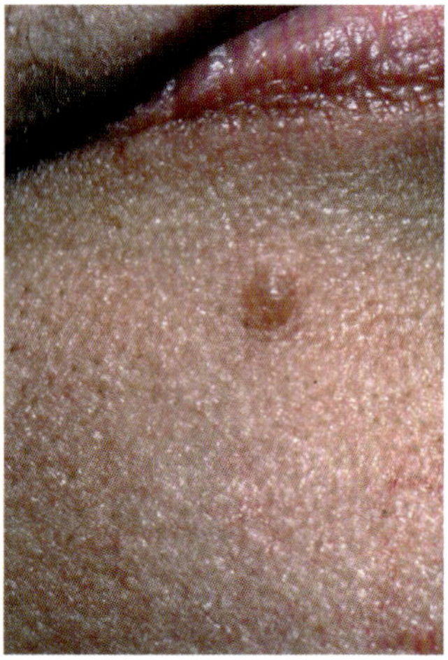

Collagenoma on the chin in multiple endocrine neoplasia type I. Photo courtesy of J.R. Toro, MD.

Age of onset

Skin findings occur as early as the mid-teens. Other manifestations are evident by age 20 in half of affected individuals, and there is virtually full penetrance by age 50 years.

Epidemiology

Unknown

Inheritance

Autosomal dominant

Chromosomal location 11q13

Gene MEN1, coding for the protein menin. The gene has 10 exons and codes for a 2.8 kb transcript.

Mutational spectrum MEN1 mutations are scattered throughout the coding sequence and include nonsense, missense, deletion, insertion and splice-site mutations.

Effect of mutation Loss of heterozygosity in multiple endocrine neoplasia type I-associated tumours suggests that the MEN1 gene is a tumour suppressor. The menin protein is a novel protein, and its function is unknown.

Diagnosis Sequence analysis of the MEN1 gene from genomic DNA

Multiple Endocrine Neoplasia Type 2B

AKA	MEN2B; multiple mucosal neuroma syndrome; Wagenmann-Froboese syndrome. Formerly called MEN3.
MIM	162300
Clinical features	Multiple mucosal neuromas, especially of the lips, tongue and conjunctiva. Tall, thin, Marfanoid habitus. Muscle weakness and wasting. Gastrointestinal symptoms due to ganglioneuromas and colonic diverticula. Increased risk of malignancy including phaeochromocytoma and medullary thyroid carcinoma.
Age of onset	First year of life
Epidemiology	Unknown
Inheritance	Autosomal dominant
Chromosomal location	10q11.2
Gene	RET, standing for *RE*arranged during *T*ransfection, is a receptor tyrosine kinase, a cell-surface molecule that transduces signals for cell growth and differentiation. The gene contains 20 exons.
Mutational spectrum	A single mutation, Met^{918}Thr in exon 16, is the only mutation identified in MEN2B affecting the catalytic core of the tyrosine kinase domain of RET.
Effect of mutation	Met^{918}Thr affects the tyrosine kinase domain of the RET oncogene
Diagnosis	Direct sequencing of genomic DNA or restriction enzyme digest to identify the codon 918 changes
Counselling issues	Half of the cases arise *de novo*, and in these situations the mutation

appears to have occurred on the paternally-derived chromosome 10. Prophylactic thyroidectomy in childhood has been proposed to reduce risk of thyroid carcinoma. Regular screening for phaeochromocytoma is recommended.

Mutations in the RET gene also cause MEN2A (MIM 171400), a disorder characterized by thyroid carcinoma, parathyroid hyperplasia and phaeochromocytoma, but with no dysmorphologic changes and no skin findings. Mutations in the RET gene are also associated with Hirschsprung disease (aganglionic megacolon; MIM 142623) and medullary thyroid carcinoma (MIM 155240).

Dyskeratosis Congenita

AKA	Zinsser-Cole-Engman syndrome
MIM	305000
Clinical features	Reticulated skin pigmentation. Atrophy. Telangiectasia. Nail dystrophy. Oral leukoplakia and other mucosal surface involvement. Thrombocytopaenia, anaemia and pancytopaenia.
Age of onset	"Dirty neck" skin changes in childhood may be the first clinical sign. The skin changes and oral malignancies begin in early adulthood. Marrow failure onset in teen years.
Epidemiology	Due to X-linked inheritance, the vast majority of cases are male
Inheritance	X-linked recessive
Chromosomal location	Xq28
Gene	DKC1, dyskerin, a ubiquitously-expressed protein. It is thought that dyskerin is a nuclear protein that is responsible for some early steps in ribosomal RNA processing. DKC1 contains 15 exons spanning at least 16 kb.
Mutational spectrum	Different missense mutations have been described in many different families. One patient has been reported with a 3′ deletion of the gene. In addition, there appears to be a common, fairly conservative, missense mutation $Ala^{353}Val$, which was seen in 11 of 21 families in one study.
Effect of mutation	Hypothesized to disrupt cell cycle, nucleolar, and telomerase functions. Non-random X-inactivation patterns can be seen in female carriers.

Diagnosis

Sequence analysis of the DKC1 gene using genomic DNA

Counselling issues

There are also autosomal recessive (MIM 224230) and autosomal dominant (MIM 127550) forms of dyskeratosis congenita, wherein the dominant form has a milder phenotype. Some sporadic affected females may actually be carriers of the X-linked recessive mutation. There is an increased risk for squamous cell cancer, oral cancers, Hodgkin disease and pancreatic adenocarcinoma. Infection, haemorrhage and malignancy often lead to demise prior to 40 years of age.

Tuberous Sclerosis

AKA

Bourneville disease

MIM

191100 (tuberous sclerosis 1; TS1); 191092 (tuberous sclerosis 2; TS2)

Clinical features

Facial angiofibroma (adenoma sebacum). Hypopigmented ash-leaf shaped macules. Shagreen patches (collagenomas). Periungual fibromas. Confetti-like hypopigmented macules. Cortical and subcortical white matter tubers (hamartomas). Infantile spasm. Seizures. Mental retardation. Calcified glial nodules. Hamartomas of cardiac tissue. Renal and adrenal angiolipomas and cysts. Retinal hamartomas and iris hypopigmentation. Pitted enamel hypoplasia.

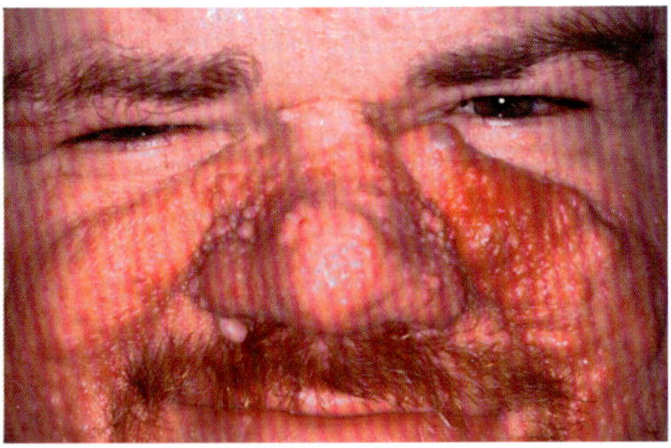

Angiofibromas in tuberous sclerosis. Photo courtesy of J.R. Toro, MD.

Age of onset

Infancy to early childhood

Epidemiology

Genetic heterogeneity exists, with some families showing linkage to chromosome 9, others to chromosome 16, and yet others to neither of these chromosomal regions, implying the existence of at least one other tuberous sclerosis locus.

Inheritance

Autosomal dominant

Chromosomal location 9q34 (TS1); 16p13.3 (TS2)

Genes TSC1 (tuberous sclerosis 1) has 23 exons and codes for hamartin, a protein containing 1164 amino acids. TSC2 (tuberous sclerosis 2) has 42 exons and produces a 5.5 kb messenger RNA. It encodes tuberin, a protein with a GAP-related domain.

Mutational spectrum Most TSC1 mutations result in a truncated protein. Truncation mutations and missense mutations are about equally represented in TSC2. The missense mutations are often located in the GAP-related domain of the gene, exons 16 and 17.

Effect of mutation Hamartin has been hypothesized to act as a tumour suppressor protein. Tuberin is hypothesized to function as a regulator of RAB5-GTP activity in endocytosis.

Diagnosis Linkage analysis can often be accomplished in appropriate families. SSCP of genomic DNA fragments, protein truncation tests and cDNA sequence analyses can be used to identify specific mutations once the determination of TSC1 versus TSC2 is made.

Counselling issues TSC1 mutations are under-represented in sporadic cases of tuberous sclerosis; these are more likely to be due to TSC2 mutations. Mutations in TSC1 account for approximately 25% of all tuberous sclerosis cases, while TSC2 mutations are found in about half of familial tuberous sclerosis. TSC2 may be more severe than TSC1, especially with respect to cognitive ability.

Cylindromatosis

AKA	Turban tumour syndrome; epithelioma adenoides cysticum; Brooke-Fordyce syndrome
MIM	132700
Clinical features	Scalp and face papules and dermal nodules which enlarge and become disfigured. Some patients have multiple trichoepitheliomas.
Age of onset	Puberty
Epidemiology	An increased frequency in Eskimos
Inheritance	Autosomal dominant
Chromosomal location	16q12-q13
Gene	Unknown
Effect of mutation	Loss of heterozygosity on 16q12-q13 in DNA obtained from the tumours as compared to constitutional (normal) DNA in the patient suggests that the gene functions as a tumour suppressor.
Diagnosis	Linkage analysis could hypothetically be performed in informative families
Counselling issues	Although the disorder is inherited in an autosomal dominant manner, a preponderance of affected females has been reported. There is a risk of malignant degeneration of the cylindromas to basal cell epithelioma.

3. Bullous Disorders

The epidermolysis bullosa (EB) disorders are grouped into Simplex, Junctional and Dystrophic types based on the level of the skin in which the blister occurs. In the Simplex types of EB, the blister occurs above the plasma membrane in the basal layer of cells. The skin heals without scarring. In Junctional forms of EB, the blister occurs within the lamina lucida. In general, the lesions are considered to be of the non-scarring type, although secondary infection of the blisters can lead to scars upon healing. In Dystrophic EB, the blister occurs below the lamina lucida within the dermis, and on healing there is scarring.

Many believe that the definitive diagnosis of EB is made by electron microscopic examination of the skin.

Epidermolysis Bullosa Simplex (EBS)

AKA

Includes the Dowling-Meara type (EB Herpetiformis), Koebner type and Weber-Cockayne type

MIM

131760 (Dowling-Meara); 131900 (Koebner); 131800 (Weber-Cockayne)

Clinical features

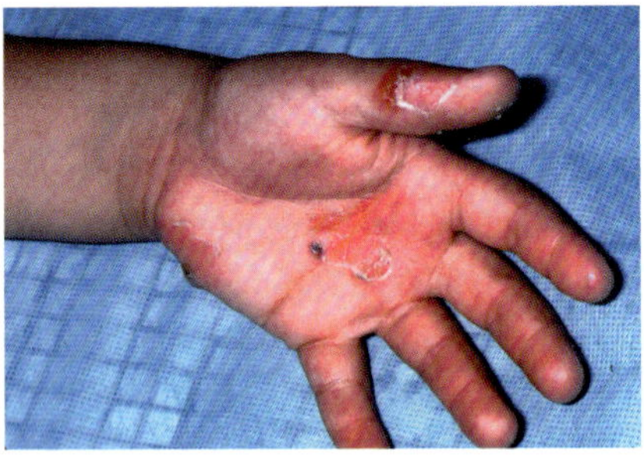

Blisters of palms and fingers in a young child with epidermolysis bullosa simplex.

Dowling-Meara

Severe blistering affecting any part of the body, often occurring in groups (herpetiformis distribution). Frequent sites include palms and soles, peri-oral area, trunk and neck. Lesions generally heal without scarring. Peri-ungual blisters may lead to nail loss. Milia. Palm and sole hyperkeratosis is common. There is often improvement of clinical features with age. In severe cases, neonatal death may ensue.

Koebner

Generalized distribution of blisters without the clustering seen in Dowling-Meara. Occasional oral, vaginal and nail involvement. Palm and sole hyperkeratosis can occur. The symptoms worsen in hot weather.

Weber-Cockayne

The blisters are distributed acrally, and are more frequent on the palms and soles than the dorsum of the hands and feet. Trauma can cause blisters on other parts of the body. The symptoms worsen in hot weather.

Age of onset

Dowling-Meara

Neonatal onset

Koebner

Onset in infancy

Weber-Cockayne

From toddler to early adolescent. Onset may occur in young men in the military when they first go on long marches.

Epidemiology

Reported in many ethnicities

Inheritance

Autosomal dominant

Transmission electron microscopy

The separation (blister) occurs above the basal or suprabasal epidermal layer. In the Dowling-Meara type, tonofilament clumping is characteristic.

Chromosomal location

12q11-13; 17q12-q21

Genes

Mutations in either of the two keratins expressed in the basal layer of the epidermis can cause EBS. KRT5, on chromosome 12, codes for keratin 5 (a type II keratin), and KRT14 (a type I keratin), on chromosome 17, codes for keratin 14. The keratin 5 and 14 proteins form heteroduplexes and higher-order complexes that generate the intermediate filament cytoskeleton to give the keratinocyte mechanical integrity. The keratin genes contain 7 or 8 exons (type I and II, respectively) in approximately 5-8 kb of genomic DNA.

Mutational spectrum

Dowling-Meara

Most cases (40%) have a point mutation in KRT14 at Arg^{125}. The changes are mostly to cysteine (Arg^{125}Cys) or to histidine (Arg^{125}His). The remainder of mutations, both in KRT5 and KRT14, cluster in the parts of the genes that code for the ends of the rod domains of the keratin protein.

Koebner

Mutations occur that affect proline residues, and the mutations are located more centrally affecting the α-helical rod domain of the keratin protein.

Weber-Cockayne

Mutations occur more frequently in KRT5 than in KRT14, but in either case the mutations cluster in the portion of the gene that codes for the head domain or the L1-2 linker segment of the protein.

There is some suggestion that the position within the protein affected by the gene mutation correlates with the severity of disease; specifically, mutations affecting the head and tail domains of the keratin protein cause more severe disease than those affecting the more central portions. In Ireland, most cases of EBS have been shown to be caused by one of three mutations: Met^{272}Arg and Asn^{193}Lys in keratin 14, and Met^{327}Tyr in keratin 5.

Effect of mutation

The presence of 50% abnormal keratin protein in the cell interferes with the assembly of normal intermediate size keratin filaments and causes the keratinocyte to become fragile.

Diagnosis

Electron microscopic analysis will confirm the specific position of the separation within the skin. Screening of genomic DNA for mutations occurring at the hot spots is the first step in mutation analysis; this is accomplished by sequencing PCR-amplified fragments from the appropriate parts of the gene. Complete genomic DNA sequence analysis should identify the remainder of mutations.

Counselling issues

Rare cases of EBS inherited in a recessive manner have been reported in the offspring of consanguineous parents who both have the disease and carry a KRT14 mutation. EBS-Ogna type (MIM 131950), reported only in Norway, is characterized by acral blisters and bruising. The gene has been mapped to 8q24. New mutation dominant cases of EBS are a frequent occurrence.

Epidermolysis Bullosa Simplex with Mottled Pigmentation

MIM

131960

Clinical features

Recurrent blistering resembling that of Koebner type (generalized distribution without clustering of lesions, see page 70) with 2-5 mm speckled hyper- and hypo-pigmented areas giving the skin a mottled appearance. Prematurely aged appearance of the skin. Mild bruisability affecting the lower extremities. Longitudinally curved nails.

Age of onset

Congenital

Inheritance

Autosomal dominant

Chromosomal location

12q11-13

Gene

KRT5, on chromosome 12, coding for keratin 5 (a type II keratin). The gene contains 8 exons.

Mutational spectrum

In two unrelated families, and one sporadic case, a C$\rightarrow$T transition at position 71 in the KRT5 gene has been found. This results in a Pro^{24}Lys change in the keratin 5 protein.

Effect of mutation

The Pro^{24}Lys mutation is hypothesized to change the physical shape of the head domain of the keratin 5 protein and cause aberration in intermediate filament protein structure and melanosome distribution. However, melanocytes appear normal in this disorder.

Diagnosis

Identification of the specific mutation causing Pro^{24}Lys can be accomplished using PCR-based allele specific detection.

Counselling issues

Ultrastructural and histological examination yields results resembling those from the other EBS subtypes.

Epidermolysis Bullosa Simplex with Muscular Dystrophy

AKA	EBS with limb-girdle muscular dystrophy
MIM	226670
Clinical features	EBS, with blistering in the neonatal period. The blistering tendency continues throughout life if the skin is traumatized. No scarring. Progressive muscular weakness of the limb-girdle type.
Age of onset	Blistering has neonatal onset; muscular weakness begins in early adulthood.
Epidemiology	Reported in 11 families to date, in Finland, South America, Germany and elsewhere
Inheritance	Autosomal recessive
Chromosomal location	8q24
Gene	PLEC1 (aka HD1), coding for plectin 1, one of the largest polypeptides known, is expressed in the inner plaques of the hemidesmosome and sarcolemma of muscle. The gene contains 32 exons extending over 32 kb. The organization of the gene is similar to that of BPAG1 which encodes bullous pemphigoid antigen 1. The amino terminus of the plectin protein has homology to the actin binding domain of the dystrophin protein family, and the carboxy terminus has homology to desmoplakin, an intermediate filament associated protein.

Mutational spectrum

Deletions (from 1 to 19 bp), duplications or insertions have been described in seven families. In half the cases, the mutations have been homozygous due to consanguinity of the parents. With rare exceptions, mutations lead to premature stop codons.

Effect of mutation

Absence of plectin, a large protein with multiple functions, is thought to impair binding of the keratin intermediate filament network to hemidesmosomes and possibly also of actin to membrane complexes.

Diagnosis

A protein truncation test (PTT) to detect mutations that result in premature termination codons will identify most mutations. Direct sequence analysis of PCR-amplified genomic fragments will detect the few remaining missense mutations.

Counselling issues

Several patients have been described with mucous airway disease including isolated blisters of the larynx or stridor. This may occur prior to the onset of muscular dystrophy. It is interesting to note that the Ogna variant of EBS also maps to 8q24, although the responsible gene has yet to be identified.

Epidermolysis Bullosa-Herlitz Type

AKA

EB letalis; junctional EB-Herlitz type; junctional EB-Herlitz-Pearson type. Non-Herlitz type also discussed.

MIM

226700

Clinical features

Severe, generalized blistering at birth. There may be congenital absence of skin. Exuberant granulation tissue, especially of the perioral and perinasal area occurs in children surviving infancy. Sloughing of the mucosa of the respiratory system can lead to obstruction and death. Shedding of the nails. Corneal erosions and corneal scarring. Dental enamel dysplasia. Balanitis in males. The bullae are considered non-scarring, although secondary infection can cause scarring as the lesions heal.

Age of onset

Congenital

Epidemiology

Many ethnic populations; consanguinity in parents is common.

Inheritance

Autosomal recessive

Transmission electron microscopy

The separation (blister) occurs above the basement membrane, within the lamina lucida at the junction of the dermis and epidermis. Absent or abnormal hemidesmosomes.

Chromosomal location

1q51 (LAMC2); 1q32 (LAMB3); 18q11.2 (LAMA3)

Genes

The anchoring filament protein, laminin-5 (aka nicein or kalinin) is composed of three polypeptides, each of which is coded for by a single gene. Mutation in both alleles of any of these three genes can lead to the disorder. LAMA3, on chromosome 18q, codes for the α-3 chain of laminin-5. LAMB3, on chromosome 1q32, codes for the β-3 chain, and LAMC2, on chromosome 1q51, codes for the γ-2 chain of laminin-5.

Mutational spectrum

All mutations to date in the Herlitz-type of junctional EB (and a very large series has been described) lead to premature termination codons and, thus, unstable mRNA that decays and is not translated into protein. The overwhelming majority of Herlitz-type cases are due to mutations in LAMB3. There are two mutational hot spots in LAMB3 resulting in the mutations Arg^{635}Stop and Arg^{42}Stop that together comprise more than half of the Junctional EB-Herlitz related LAMB3 alleles. In LAMA3, a hotspot, Arg^{650}Stop, was described in three out of four families. LAMC2 mutations, on the other hand, appear to be different in each family, with the exception of Arg^{95}Stop which has been reported more than once.

In a group of patients with a non-Herlitz-type clinical phenotype of junctional EB, there were some who also had mutations in LAMB3 or LAMC2. Whereas mutations leading to premature termination of protein translation cause the Herlitz-type, this group of non-Herlitz type patients were found to have a premature termination mutation on one allele, while the other carried a missense (and presumably, milder) mutation, or missense mutations occurred on both alleles. The same LAMB3 hotspots are found in both the Herlitz and non-Herlitz types, and account for about 25% of all the mutant LAMB3 alleles in this type of non-Herlitz junctional EB.

Effect of mutation

In Herlitz-type, absence of functional laminin-5 protein, a major anchoring filament protein, appears to lead to fragility and separation of the epidermis from the dermis. The milder phenotype of the Non-Herlitz type may be due to the presence of at least some laminin-5 protein, however abnormal, associated with the missense mutations.

Diagnosis

PCR-amplification and sequence analysis of amplified genomic DNA or PCR-based allele-specific assays to identify the presence of the common mutations in the LAMB3 gene should be accomplished first. If this analysis is negative, genomic DNA sequence analysis of the rest of the LAMB3 gene should be performed, and, if negative, the LAMA3 and LAMC2 genes can be screened by the same method.

Counselling issues

Herlitz-type junctional EB is frequently lethal in infancy, often due to sepsis or airway obstruction. However, there are several reports of patients surviving to their teen years.

Junctional Epidermolysis Bullosa with Pyloric Atresia

AKA

JEB-PA, considered a type of non-Herlitz junctional EB

MIM

226730

Clinical features

Congenital pyloric atresia. Gastrointestinal symptoms, including membranous pyloric antrum obstruction, diarrhoea, protein-losing gastroenteropathy and gastric dilatation. Pyelonephrosis. Aplasia cutis congenita is seen consistently. Axillary pterygia. Perioral blisters. Erosions of oral mucosa, upper oesophagus and cornea. Ectropion. Ear and nose deformities. Distal limb contraction (arthrogryposis). Ureterovesical junction stenosis.

Age of onset

Infancy

Epidemiology

Rare

Inheritance

Autosomal recessive

Immunofluorescence microscopy

Absence of staining with antibody against the hemidesmosomal integrin $\alpha6/\beta4$

Chromosomal location

17q11-qter; chr 2

Gene

Integrins are transmembrane glycoprotein receptors involved in cell-cell and cell-matrix adhesion. The molecules are heterodimers, containing one α and one β subunit. Integrin $\alpha6/\beta4$, expressed in basal keratinocytes, is restricted to the ventral surface apposed to the basement membrane zone and is associated with hemidesmosomes in both stratified and transitional epithelia. The gene for the β subunit of integrin $\alpha6/\beta4$ (ITGB4) is located on chromosome 17 and consists of 41 exons spanning 36 kb of genomic DNA. The gene for the α-subunit (ITGA6) is on chromosome 2, and consists of 27 exons, one of which (exon 5B) is an additional exon present only in certain tissue-specific alternate transcripts. Mutation of both alleles of either subunit gene leads to the JEB-PA phenotype.

Mutational spectrum

Most mutations described result in a premature termination codon and lack of translation of the integrin component protein.

Effect of mutation

The clinical manifestations of JEB-PA suggest that this integrin has tissue-specific roles in both skin and gastrointestinal tract. The pyloric lumen appears to be replaced by loose connective tissue. Mutations are thought to affect the integrity of the basement membrane and hemidesmosomes and also normal control of fibrosis during wound healing.

Diagnosis

Sequence analysis of cDNA prepared from mRNA using reverse transcriptase-polymerase chain reaction (RT-PCR) or PCR amplification of each exon of the laminin chain genes from genomic DNA, followed by heteroduplex analysis and direct sequencing of the PCR products, will identify the mutations. When the specific DNA mutations are unknown, foetal skin biopsy has been used for diagnosis. Ultrasound examination of the foetus may identify duodenal atresia. However this is not a dependable diagnostic approach.

Counselling issues

Death occurs in infancy, usually due to pyloric abnormality or other gastrointestinal complications. Ultrasound examination of an at-risk foetus may reveal gastric dilatation associated with the disease and be a basis for pre-natal diagnosis. Occasional non-lethal cases have been reported.

Generalized Atrophic Benign Epidermolysis Bullosa

AKA	GABEB; epidermolysis bullosa-Disentis type; GABEB is considered a type of non-Herlitz junctional EB
MIM	226650
Clinical features	Blisters at birth but decreasing in frequency with age. Scarring does not occur, although blisters heal with atrophy. Nail dystrophy. Scarring alopecia of the scalp, eyebrows, eyelashes and pubic/axillary hair. Blisters of mucosal surfaces. Dental enamel defects and carious teeth.
Age of onset	Birth
Epidemiology	Described in patients of Austrian or Dutch background
Inheritance	Autosomal recessive
Transmission electron microscopy	Cleavage within the lamina lucida. Abnormal or decreased numbers of hemidesmosomes.
Chromosomal location	10q24.3
Gene	BPAG2, coding for bullous pemphigoid antigen 2 (more appropriately called COL17A1, coding for the α-1 chain of collagen 17). The gene contains 56 exons in 52 kb of genomic DNA.
Mutational spectrum	The majority of mutations result in premature termination codons with a few splice-site and missense mutations reported. It appears that there is no phenotypic difference between those cases of GABEB caused by two premature termination mutations or those

due to a mutation causing premature termination of translation on one allele and a missense mutation on the other.

Effect of mutation

Type 17 collagen is a homotrimer composed of three α-1 chains. Mutation results in a deficiency of the collagen 17 component of the hemidesmosomal structure.

Diagnosis

CSGE of genomic DNA, followed by sequence analysis of exons with abnormal patterns, and heteroduplex analysis have been used to identify mutations in the very large collagen genes.

Counselling issues

Although the disorder is inherited in an autosomal recessive manner, a dominantly-inherited mutation causing a glycine substitution in type 17 collagen has been reported in one large family. The proband with GABEB carried the glycine substituted allele and a premature termination mutation on the second COL17A1 allele. The family members with only the glycine substitution and no other COL17A1 mutation had markedly abnormal dentition and enamel pitting, but no blisters. The clinical phenotype of GABEB has also been described in patients with laminin-5 gene mutations.

Dystrophic Epidermolysis Bullosa, Recessive Type

AKA

Recessive epidermolysis bullosa dystrophica (REBD), includes Hallopeau-Siemens type, Inversa type, Mitis type and Localized type

MIM

226600

Clinical features

There are several clinical subtypes of REBD, although all are so far associated with mutation in COL7A1 (see below).

Hallopeau-Siemens type

Characterized by serous or haemorrhagic blisters involving hands, feet, elbows, knees, mucosal surfaces, conjunctiva and corneas. Blisters spread and self-enlarge. Ulcerations and erosions heal slowly and with scarring. Milia. Pruritis. Loss of nail plates. Digital fusion and auto-amputation result in the classic mitten deformity. Occasionally, congenital absence of skin. Ectropion. Dysphagia. Oesophageal webs and stricture. Malnutrition due to difficulty in swallowing. Microstomia. Defective dental enamel. Limb contractures.

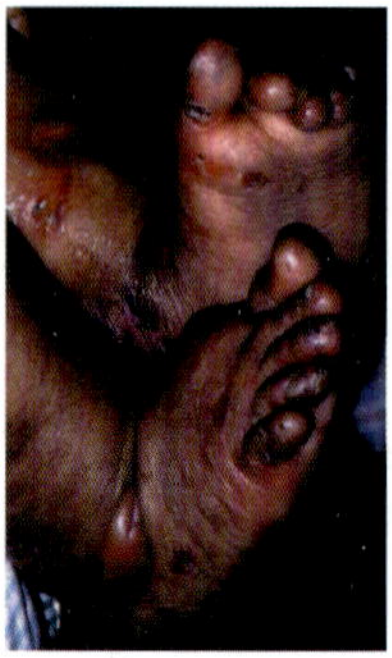

Blisters and loss of nail plates in the Hallopeau-Siemens type of recessive dystrophic epidermolysis bullosa in an infant.

Mitis type

Similar to Hallopeau-Siemens, but milder and usually without the mitten deformities.

Localized type

Blisters are restricted to the extremities.

Inversa type

Generalized blistering of infancy becomes limited to flexures, groin and trunk with age. These patients have severe oral and oesophageal involvement.

Age of onset

Birth or early infancy

Epidemiology

Worldwide

Inheritance

Autosomal recessive

Transmission electron microscopy

The blister occurs within the dermis. There are absent or decreased numbers of anchoring fibrils.

Chromosomal location

3p21

Gene

COL7A1, coding for the pro-α-1 chain of type VII collagen.
The gene contains 118 exons, the largest number in any published gene to date, and covers 32 kb of genomic DNA. Type VII collagen is the major (perhaps exclusive) component of the anchoring fibrils that connect the lamina densa to the papillary dermis.

Mutational spectrum

Over 90 mutations in more than 100 families have been characterized. The vast majority of patients with Hallopeau-Siemens type have a mutation on both alleles that results in a premature truncation codon. In the Mitis form, the mutations are frequently missense or in-frame deletions in one or both alleles.

Several recurrent mutations have been identified, the most frequent being Arg^{578}Stop and ^{7786}delG.

Effect of mutation

In patients with Hallopeau-Siemens type REBD, the premature truncation codon leads to accelerated decay of mRNA and very low production (if any) of type VII collagen. No anchoring fibrils are formed. Mutations in the Mitis form result in the production of collagen protein with abnormal conformation, assembly or packing of fibrils (some of which can be detected ultrastructurally). Too few mutations in the other subtypes of REBD have been identified to allow further genotype/phenotype correlation.

Diagnosis

PCR-amplification of exons from genomic DNA, followed by heteroduplex scanning of the PCR products. For patients with homozygous mutations, DNA from the patient and a control individual who is unaffected are mixed together before performing the heteroduplex analysis. Alternatively, DGGE or SSCP has been used.

Counselling issues

Patients have a very high risk of developing squamous cell carcinoma in the areas where there has been repeated blistering and scarring. The squamous cell carcinomas develop in early adulthood.

Dystrophic Epidermolysis Bullosa, Dominant Type

AKA

Dominant epidermolysis bullosa dystrophica (DEBD), includes Cockayne-Touraine type, Pasini type, Pretibial type, Bart syndrome and Pruriginosa type

MIM

131750 (Pasini type); 132000 (Bart syndrome);
604129 (Pruriginosa type); 131800 (Cockayne-Touraine type);
131850 (Pretibial type)

Clinical features

There are several clinical subtypes of DEBD, although all are so far associated with mutation in COL7A1 (see below).

Pasini type

Characterized by widespread blistering. Blisters heal with scarring and milia. Nail dystrophy. Oral mucosal involvement. Characteristic Pasini papules are small, albulopapuloid, white, scar-like lesions that appear spontaneously, unassociated with prior blisters.

Cockayne-Touraine type

Blisters localized to the extremities (over the elbows, knees, fingers and toes) which heal with scarring and milia. Oral involvement may occur.

Bart syndrome

Absence of skin over the tibias. Blisters affect skin and mucous membranes.

Pruriginosa type

Characterized by skin fragility, blisters and scar formation with intense itching. Nail dystrophy. Lichenified lesions.

Pretibial type

Epidermolysis bullosa restricted to the pretibial areas, where blisters then develop into prurigo-like hyperkeratotic lesions. Nail dystrophy. Albulopapuloid lesions. Scars.

Age of onset

Pasini

Blistering occurs at birth or soon after, with the Pasini papules usually developing around the age of adolescence.

Cockayne-Touraine

Infancy or early childhood

Bart syndrome

Birth

Pruriginosa

Childhood to early adulthood

Epidemiology

Worldwide

Inheritance

Autosomal dominant

Transmission electron microscopy

The blister occurs below the lamina densa in the dermis. The anchoring fibrils are thin and reduced in number.

Chromosomal location

3p21

Gene

COL7A1, coding for the pro-α-1 chain of type VII collagen. The gene contains 118 exons, the largest number in any published gene to date, and covers 32 kb of genomic DNA. Type VII collagen is the major (perhaps exclusive) component of the anchoring fibrils that connect the lamina densa to the papillary dermis.

Mutational spectrum

Nearly all mutations causing the DEBD result in replacement of a glycine residue in the pro-α-1 chain of type VII collagen with another amino acid. Gly2043Arg represents a common mutation found in patients from many ethnic backgrounds. Glycine substitutions in exon 73 have been found in Cockayne-Touraine, Pasini and Bart types of DEBD. The clinical differences between these types may result from the specific location of the glycine substitution caused by the exon 73 mutation.

Effect of mutation

The glycine substitutions all affect residues in the collagenous domain of the type VII collagen molecule. The mutated polypeptides are of normal length and assemble into the usual triple-helix of collagen molecules. However, the presence of another amino acid, where glycine should be, is destabilizing to the helix resulting in anchoring fibrils that are thin and reduced in number.

Diagnosis

PCR-amplification of exons from genomic DNA, followed by heteroduplex scanning of the PCR products. Specifically, double-stranded heteroduplexes that form between the mutant DNA strand and the normal DNA strand can be distinguished from homoduplexes (two strands having the same sequence). Alternatively, DGGE or SSCP has been used.

Counselling issues

Although glycine substitutions are characteristic of DEBD, not all glycine substitutions exert a dominant phenotypic effect. There are cases of patients with REBD where one or both alleles carry glycine substitutions, but the heterozygous parents of the affected children are clinically normal.

In patients with a mild phenotype and clinically normal parents, the temptation is to assume that the case is the result of a new dominant mutation. However, only a single *de novo* dominant mutation in COL7A1 has been confirmed to date. It is much more likely that a new, sporadic case in a family is due to recessive inheritance.

4

4. Pigmentary Disorders

Haemochromatosis

MIM 235200

Clinical features Grey, brown or bronze colouration to the skin, including genitalia and oral mucosa. Alopecia and hypotrichosis. Xerosis. Nail changes. Untreated patients can develop heart and liver failure, arthropathy and diabetes mellitus.

Age of onset In males, onset occurs when middle-aged; in females, it occurs after the menopause

Epidemiology Haemochromatosis affects 1:300 Caucasians of Northern European origin. Approximately 25% of Caucasians and 15% of Hispanics carry one copy of the $His^{63}Asp$ allele. The $Cys^{282}Tyr$ allele is carried by 8% of Caucasians, 3% of Hispanics and 2% of African-Americans.

Inheritance Autosomal dominant

Chromosomal location 6p21.3

Gene HFE (at one time called HLA-H), a major histocompatibility complex (MHC) Class I-like gene

Mutational spectrum Most $C^{282}Y$ homozygotes (98%) have clinical disease, compared to only 38% of $Cys^{282}Tyr/His^{63}Asp$. The $Cys^{282}Tyr$ allele is much more penetrant than the $His^{63}Asp$ allele; in fact, $His^{63}Asp$ homozygotes very rarely have haemochromatosis.

Effect of mutation The $Cys^{282}Tyr$ mutation has been shown to completely prevent the association of the HFE protein with the transferrin receptor. $His^{63}Asp$ may interfere with the affinity of the transferrin receptor for transferrin.

Diagnosis

High serum transferrin saturation with increased fasting ferritin. Molecular diagnosis can be accomplished by screening for common HFE mutations using genomic DNA.

Counselling issues

Genetic heterogeneity exists, as there are families whose disease phenotype does not map to chromosome 6p and in whom no HFE mutations have been found. There is an increased risk for hepatic cancer which can be prevented by appropriate treatment of the haemochromatosis.

Hypomelanosis of Ito

AKA

Incontinentia pigmenti achromians (IP1)

MIM

146150

Clinical features

Whorls, streaks and patches of hypopigmentation, in a negative pattern as compared to the hyperpigmentation seen in incontinentia pigmenti. Rare dental anomalies, including abnormally-shaped teeth. Mental retardation. Seizures. Cataract. Iris coloboma.

Age of onset

Congenital, but may become more noticeable throughout early childhood years

Epidemiology

Diagnosed in 1:8000-10,000 unselected patients at a Spanish children's hospital

Inheritance

Heterogeneous disorder. Most patients have chromosomal mosaicism (two cell lines with different genetic/chromosome complements), but autosomal dominant inheritance has been described in some families.

Chromosome findings

Chromosomal mosaicism (two different cell lines) in epidermal keratinocytes. No chromosome abnormality observed in cultured lymphocytes. The mosaicism can consist of a mixture of diploid and triploid cells, or a line with a chromosomal deletion, translocation or supernumerary chromosome, and also a normal line. Either autosomes or sex chromosomes can be involved in the mosaicism.

Effect of genetic anomaly

It is hypothesized that hypomelanosis of Ito, a heterogeneous condition, is a cutaneous marker of somatic mosaicism. In some cases, the condition may be due to loss of function, in one line of cells, of genes involved in pigment formation.

Diagnosis

The absence of the inflammatory stage of the lesions during the neonatal period helps differentiate hypomelanosis of Ito from incontinentia pigmenti. Chromosome analysis of cultured keratinocytes should allow identification of the mosaic chromosome complement.

Counselling issues

Although the majority of cases are probably due to somatic mosaicism, it should be kept in mind that there have been several reports of parent-offspring transmission, without observable chromosomal anomalies, that suggest autosomal dominant inheritance.

Incontinentia Pigmenti

AKA IP2

MIM 308310

Clinical features Affected females have a progressive vesicular and erythematous eruption, which soon becomes verrucous and hyperkeratotic, and subsequently pigmented, often in a swirling, marble cake distribution. In the final stage, the lesions become atrophic. Adolescents and adults may be left with areas of linear and reticular hypopigmentation. Rarely, alopecia and hypodontia occur, as well as microcephaly and mental retardation, and vascular and retinal pigmentary abnormalities.

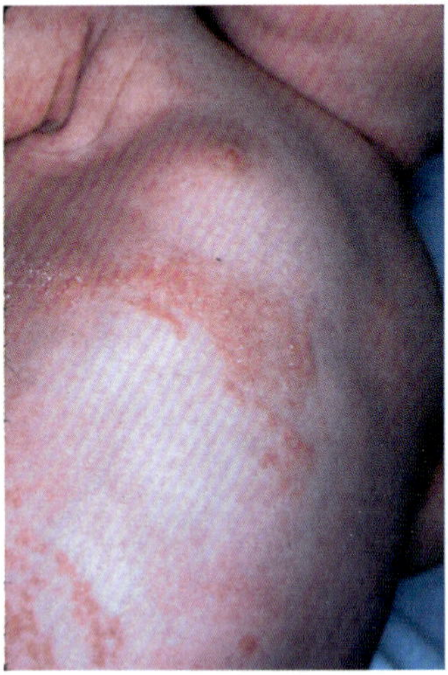

Multiple vescicles following lines of Blaschko in the early stage of incontinentia pigmenti.
Photo courtesy of J.R. Toro, MD.

Age of onset Neonatal period

Epidemiology Virtually restricted to females, as IP2 is thought to be lethal in males

Inheritance X-linked dominant

Chromosomal location Xq28

Gene Unknown

Effect of mutation It has been hypothesized that evolution of skin lesions represents death of those cells that carry the mutant IP2 gene on the X-chromosome, and replacement by cells carrying the normal, active X-chromosome.

Diagnosis Nearly all affected females have completely skewed patterns of X-inactivation in peripheral leukocytes. In familial cases, linkage studies to identify the disease-carrying X-chromosome may be used to perform prenatal diagnosis.

Counselling issues It is now thought that the sporadic form of IP2, sometimes called IP1 (MIM 308300), is actually hypomelanosis of Ito (see page 96). In cases of IP2 resulting from a new mutation, paternally-derived mutations are reported to occur twice as often as maternally-derived mutations. A high rate of spontaneous abortion occurs in women carrying the IP2 gene, probably due to loss of affected male foetuses.

McCune-Albright Syndrome

AKA	Polyostotic fibrous dysplasia with café-au-lait spots; Albright syndrome
MIM	174800
Clinical features	Large café-au-lait spots with irregular margins, usually on one side of the body and not crossing the midline. Polyostotic fibrous dysplasia (bone lucencies that distort bone structure). Hyperthyroidism. Parathyroidism. Prolactinaemia. Cushing Syndrome. Precocious puberty in females. Acromegaly.
Age of onset	Congenital or in infancy
Epidemiology	Rare
Inheritance	Sporadic, due to somatic mosaicism for a post-zygotic mutation
Chromosomal location	20q13.2
Gene	GNAS1, coding for guanine nucleotide-binding protein (Gs, stimulatory). The protein is a heterotrimer.
Mutational spectrum	Activating mutations lead to constitutive activation of the gene. Mutations may be seen in DNA from one cell type (e.g. blood leukocytes) but not in others (e.g. clinically normal skin). Missense mutations affecting the Arg^{201} residue (encoded by exon 8 of the gene) have been described in several patients.
Effect of mutation	The mutations lead to activation of the GNAS1 protein and affect cellular hormone sensitivities.

Diagnosis

Both SSCP and genomic DNA sequence analysis are used to identify mutations

Counselling issues

GNAS1 mutations are also seen in autosomal dominant pseudohypoparathyroidism IA (Albright hereditary osteodystrophy). Patients with McCune-Albright syndrome have an increased risk of developing pituitary adenomas and possibly breast cancer. There can be malignant degeneration of the bony lesions. Radiotherapy to these lesions may increase the frequency of malignant changes.

Carney Complex

AKA

NAME syndrome (*N*aevi; *A*trial myxoma; *M*yxoid neurofibromata; *E*philides); LAMB syndrome (*L*entigines; *A*trial myxoma; *M*ucocutaneous myxoma; *B*lue naevi)

MIM

160980

Clinical features

Cutaneous pigmented lesions over the entire body, including lips, mucosal surfaces and conjunctiva. Lesions can be brown-black, blue or freckles (ephilides). Myxoid cutaneous tumours of many types develop on any skin surface. Atrial myxomas and myxomas of other cardiac sites. Cushing syndrome. Acromegaly. Breast fibroadenoma. Thyroid lesions. Myxomas of the eyelid.

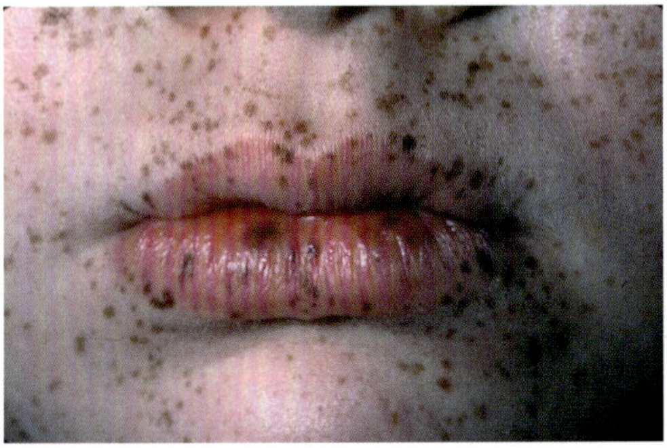

Multiple pigmented macules in the perioral area and lips in a young woman with Carney complex. Photo courtesy of J.R. Toro, MD.

Age of onset

Early childhood

Inheritance

Autosomal dominant

Chromosomal location

2p16; 17q2

Gene

Unknown

Effect of mutation

The Carney gene on 2p is hypothesized to have a dominant (possibly gain of function) effect leading to tumour formation, and may be involved in regulation of genomic stability of dividing cells.

Diagnosis

Linkage analysis in informative families can differentiate between chromosome 2 and chromosome 17 loci, and identify affected individuals.

Counselling issues

Increased risk of malignancy, including myxoid liposarcoma, adrenocortical carcinoma and various other rare tumours (subcutaneous myxoid neurofibroma, nasopharyngeal schwannoma and large-cell calcifying Sertoli cell tumours).

Neurofibromatosis 1

AKA

NF1, von Recklinghausen disease

MIM

162200

Clinical features

Multiple café-au-lait spots, neurofibromas and axillary and groin freckling. Dusky, dark cast to the skin. Lisch nodules (iris hamartomas) seen on slit-lamp exam post-puberty. Plexiform neurofibromas which can be debilitating and disfiguring. Scoliosis. Optic pathway and brainstem gliomas. Astrocytomas. Cognitive impairment in some patients. Pseudoarthrosis. Sphenoid dysplasia. Macrocephaly.

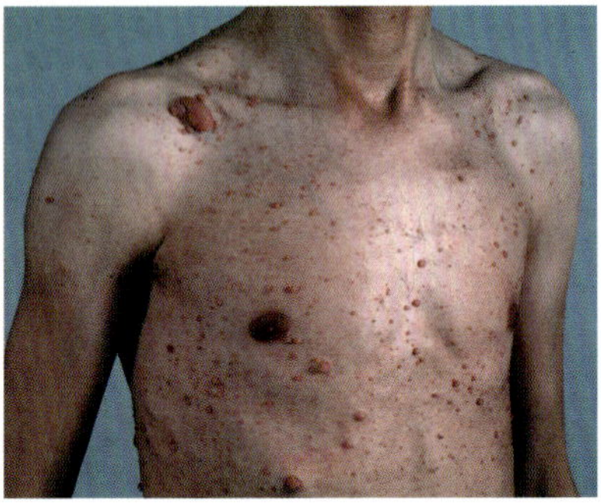

Cutaneous neurofibromas in neurofibromatosis 1. Photo courtesy of Dilys Parry, Ph.D.

Age of onset

Café-au-lait spots are present in childhood, although they may increase in number and size over time. Axillary and groin freckling occurs by puberty.

Epidemiology

Perhaps the most common of the important autosomal dominant disorders, affecting 1:3000 persons. The disease is prevalent in all ethnic groups. New mutation cases are common and more than 80% are of paternal origin.

Inheritance

Autosomal dominant

Chromosomal location 17q11.2

Gene NF1, coding for a 2818 amino acid protein named neurofibromin. The gene spans 335 kb, has more than 49 exons and produces at least three major alternative splicing products. There are other unrelated genes embedded within intron 27b of the NF1 gene.

Mutational spectrum There are only a few relative hotspots for mutation, with the remaining mutations occurring throughout the gene. A $C^{5839}T$ change, leading to $Arg^{1947}Stop$ in exon 31, is the most common of these.

Effect of mutation Most NF1 mutations predict inactivation of the neurofibromin protein, supporting haplo-insufficiency as the disease-causing mechanism for some features of the disease, but loss of heterozygosity may be the factor in NF1-associated tumour development. The function of the NF1 protein is mostly unknown, except for its interaction with Ras as a negative regulator of the Ras signalling pathway.

Diagnosis Linkage studies in appropriate families can be performed. Direct sequence analysis of genomic DNA is a large task, but is available clinically.

Counselling issues Segmental NF1, where clinical manifestations are limited to a particular area of the body, is probably caused by somatic mutation leading to tissue mosaicism. Individuals with segmental NF1 can have children with classic NF1, implying that the mosaicism involves progenitors of the germ cells in these individuals.

There is an increased risk for malignancy including various central nervous system tumours (e.g. malignant peripheral nerve sheath tumour, rhabdomyosarcoma and leukaemia), which are often asymptomatic. The role of screening (neuro-imaging) for optic pathway and other central nervous system tumours in asymptomatic children is controversial. Current recommendations are to screen using an ophthalmologic examination protocol. Treatment of the small cutaneous neurofibromas is usually for cosmetic purposes only, although very large lesions can compromise function and thus may be removed. Additionally, there is some risk for malignant transformation.

Because of the great intrafamilial variability in disease expression and severity, counselling families is problematic.

Neurofibromatosis 2

AKA

NF2, bilateral acoustic neurofibromatosis, central neurofibromatosis

MIM

101000

Clinical features

Café-au-lait spots in about half of patients, but rarely more than five (as seen in NF1). Peripheral nerve tumours (usually schwannomas, but sometimes neurofibromas) in 50-60% of affected individuals. Few have more than ten skin tumours. Bilateral eighth cranial nerve tumours (acoustic neuromas, aka vestibular schwannomas), other cranial nerve schwannomas, spinal nerve schwannomas, spinal meningiomas and ependymomas. Juvenile posterior subcapsular or cortical cataracts in 60-70% of carefully examined patients. Hearing loss and deafness.

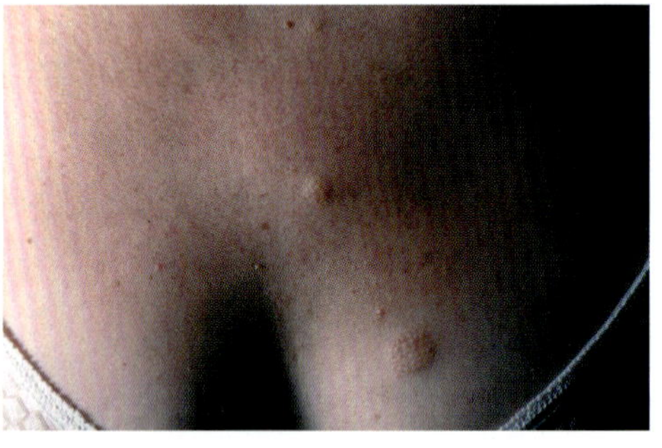

Peripheral schwannoma on the breast of a young woman with neurofibromatosis 2. Photo courtesy of Dilys Parry, Ph.D.

Age of onset

Mean age of onset is 21.5 years. Cataracts may be apparent on examination before symptoms of cranial and spinal tumours are evident, and are congenital in a small proportion of patients.

Epidemiology

1:33,000-40,500. Approximately 50% of NF2 cases are due to new mutations, where there is no family history of the disease. There may be a maternal effect on severity, in which patients who inherited their NF2 mutation from their mother have an earlier age of onset (late teens).

Inheritance Autosomal dominant

Chromosomal location 22q11.21-q13.1

Gene NF2, which has 17 exons and codes for the merlin (aka schwannomin) protein. Merlin shows homology to the ezrin-radixin-moesin class of proteins which link cytoskeleton proteins to membranes.

Mutational spectrum Half of NF2 patients have point mutations, and one-third have large deletions. A preponderance of mutations occur in the first 13 exons. Mutations causing truncation of the protein are associated with more severe clinical disease.

Effect of mutation Loss of the wild type allele in NF2-associated tumours supports the hypothesis that the protein product of NF2 functions as a tumour-suppressor.

Diagnosis Linkage studies in appropriate families. DNA screening tests, including SSCP or DGGE, can be used to identify exons with abnormal migration patterns, followed by direct sequencing.

Counselling issues NF2 is not really a genodermatosis, but is included here to clarify the differences between NF1 and NF2 that are sometimes overlooked because of the similarity in name. Gadolinium-enhanced magnetic resonance imaging (MRI) is used to show small, asymptomatic acoustic neuromas. Mosaicism (somatic mutation) is relatively common in NF2, estimated to occur in up to 15% of index cases.

Peutz-Jeghers Syndrome

AKA	Hamartomatous intestinal polyposis; Peutz-Touraine-Jehgers
MIM	175200
Clinical features	Dark pigmented macules on the lips, buccal mucosa, finger, palms and soles. Multiple hamartomatous polyps of the entire gastrointestinal tract, but jejunal polyps are seen most consistently.
Age of onset	Infancy to early childhood
Inheritance	Autosomal dominant
Chromosomal location	19p13.3
Gene	STK11, coding for a serine/threonine protein kinase II. The gene is 23 kb long and contains 9 exons.
Mutational spectrum	Mutations include intragenic rearrangements and deletions, and nonsense and splice site mutations leading to premature truncation of the protein product. Rarely, missense mutations have been described.
Effect of mutations	STK11 probably functions as a tumour suppressor gene, as evidenced by loss of heterozygosity in tumours compared to constitutional DNA in patients with Peutz-Jeghers syndrome.
Diagnosis	Sequence analysis of genomic DNA
Counselling issues	Gastrointestinal complications, including pain, intussusception and prolapse are frequent. There is a significantly elevated risk for gastrointestinal cancer, but also for gynaecological and breast cancer in women, and testicular cancer in men.

Waardenburg Syndrome (WS) (Types I, II, III and IV)

AKA

WS1; WS2; WS3 (aka Klein-Waardenburg syndrome); WS4 (aka Waardenburg-Shah syndrome)

MIM

193500 (WS1); 193510 (Ws2); 148820 (WS3); 277580 (WS4)

Clinical features

WS1

Partial albinism. White forelock and eyelashes. Premature greying. Heterochromia iridis. Hypoplastic iris stroma. Albinotic fundus. Cochlear deafness. Wide nasal bridge and short philtrum. Dystopia canthorum (laterally displaced inner canthi resulting in short palpebral fissures).

WS2

Similar to WS1 but without the dystopia canthorum.

WS3

Features described for WS1. Limb abnormalities. Musculoskeletal hypoplasia. Flexion contractures. Fusion of carpal bones and syndactyly. Some patients have neurological involvement with microcephaly and mental retardation.

WS4

No albinotic skin and no deafness. Gastrointestinal abnormalities similar to Hirschsprung disease (intestinal obstruction and microcolon). Dilated proximal ileum and collapsed distal ileum and colon.

Age of onset

Usually evident in childhood

Epidemiology

WS has been described in many populations and accounts for

1-2% of deafness in the general population. WS1 is the leading cause of deafness in South Australia.

Inheritance

WS1, WS2 and WS3 are autosomal dominant conditions, while WS4 is autosomal recessive.

Chromosomal location

2q35 (WS1 and WS3); 3p14.1-p12.3 (WS2); 22q13 (SOX10), 20q13 (EDN3) or 13q22 (EDNRB) (WS4)

Genes

PAX3 (WS1 and WS3) has 3 exons and encodes a DNA-binding protein expressed during neurogenesis. Mutations in the mouse homologue of human PAX3 cause the *splotch* phenotype in mice.

MITF (WS2) a 9-exon gene. The gene product is thought to be involved in mediating melanocyte differentiation by trans-activating the gene for tyrosinase, a key enzyme in melanogenesis.

SOX10 (WS4) a member of a gene family related to the testis-determining gene, SRY. It is also found mutated in some Hirschsprung disease patients.

EDNRB and EDN3 (WS4) endothelin-B receptor gene and its ligand, involved in the development of neural-crest derived cell lineages. Mutations have also been found in Hirschsprung disease patients.

Mutational spectrum

Most PAX3 mutations are private (observed in only one family) and occur throughout the coding sequence. PAX3 mutations account for most WS1 cases, and some WS3 cases. Mutations in MITF include deletions and insertions leading to premature truncation of the resultant protein. Also missense and nonsense mutations have been described. Mutations in SOX10 include nonsense mutations and small insertions/deletions. EDN3 and EDNRB mutations are mostly homozygous changes and include substitutions/deletions, and missense and nonsense mutations.

Effect of mutation

The mutations are predicted to interfere with normal development of neural crest derived tissues or to affect the process of melanocyte differentiation.

Diagnosis

Linkage studies in appropriate families. Direct genomic DNA sequence analysis of gene implicated by clinical features and/or linkage studies. For WS1, the efficient strategy is to first screen PAX3, and for WS2, MITF. In WS patients who also have Hirschsprung disease, the SOX10, EDN3 and EDNRB genes are better candidates.

Counselling issues

Hirschsprung disease is associated with WS, and patients should be evaluated for symptoms of the disorder. Cleft lip/palate is sometimes seen in WS1 and WS2. Hearing loss and heterochromia are more common in WS2 than WS1. Some WS2 families do not map to chromosome 3, and are considered WS2B type; the chromosomal location for this group has yet to be defined. MITF mutations are also found in some cases of ocular albinism with sensorineural deafness (MIM 103470).

Oculocutaneous Albinism Type I

AKA OCA1, tyrosinase negative albinism

MIM 203100

Clinical features Albinism with white skin, white hair, eyebrows and eyelashes. Eyes are usually light coloured. Nystagmus. Photophobia. Decreased visual acuity.

Age of onset Congenital

Epidemiology Frequently observed in populations where there are consanguineous marriages or inbreeding, or in population isolates. Tyrosinase negative and tyrosinase positive albinism were found to be equally frequent in England. OCA1 occurs in 1:10,000 in Northern Ireland and 1:35,000 in British Columbia (where tyrosinase negative OCA was twice as frequent as tyrosinase positive OCA). OCA1 is uncommon in African-American and African people.

Inheritance Autosomal recessive

Chromosomal location 11q14-q21

Gene TYR, coding for the enzyme tyrosinase. The gene contains 5 exons and spans over 50 kb.

Mutational spectrum Most mutations are missense and there are a wide variety and number of mutant alleles. Different alleles may account for the variation in clinical phenotype, including yellow albinism. Mutations tend to cluster in four areas of the gene: sequences that code for the copper A and copper B binding sites, and in exons 1 and 4.

Effect of mutation

TYR mutations cause greatly decreased or absent activity of the enzyme, tyrosinase, which is involved in the conversion of tyrosine to melanin.

Diagnosis

Sequence analysis of genomic DNA

Counselling issues

Patients have an increased risk to develop sun-induced skin cancers due to their decreased pigment. Although rare, malignant melanoma can occur and is likely to be of the amelanotic type.

Oculocutaneous Albinism Type II

AKA	OCA2, tyrosinase positive albinism
MIM	203200
Clinical features	Albinism, nystagmus and visual loss. Iris colour is blue-grey or darker. In black-skinned races, patients with OCA2 have yellow coloured hair.
Age of onset	Congenital. Some pigment may accumulate over time.
Epidemiology	Tyrosinase positive OCA is the most prevalent type of albinism in the world. The frequency is 1:36,000 in the United States, 1:10,000 in African-Americans and about 1:2000 in Africa.
Inheritance	Autosomal recessive
Chromosomal location	15q11.2-q12
Gene	OCA2 (aka P), homologous to the mouse pink-eyed dilution locus, *P*. The gene encodes a melanosome membrane protein and consists of 25 exons.
Mutational spectrum	Among South African blacks, a deletion encompassing exon 1 causes OCA2 in more than 75% of the patients. A 2.7 kb deletion accounts for most of the OCA2 in Tanzania. There are also many missense mutations.
Effect of mutation	It is thought that the OCA2 (or P) gene codes for a tyrosine transporter, thus mutations would inhibit the transport of tyrosine across the membrane of the melanosome.
Diagnosis	Direct sequencing of genomic DNA

Counselling issues

Some patients with tyrosinase positive OCA have mutations in the TYR gene, so there is clearly clinical overlap between the two types. Negroids with OCA2 who have pigmented ephilides have a lower risk of developing skin cancer than those without ephilides.

Hermansky-Pudlak Syndrome

MIM

203300

Clinical features

Oculocutaneous albinism (which may be variable in severity). Platelet storage pool deficiency leading to bleeding diathesis and lysosomal accumulation of ceroid lipofuscin. Increased freckling. Multiple melanocytic naevi. Congenital nystagmus. Easy bruising. Pulmonary fibrosis in patients with HPS1 mutations and granulomatous colitis in 10-20% of all Hermansky-Pudlak patients.

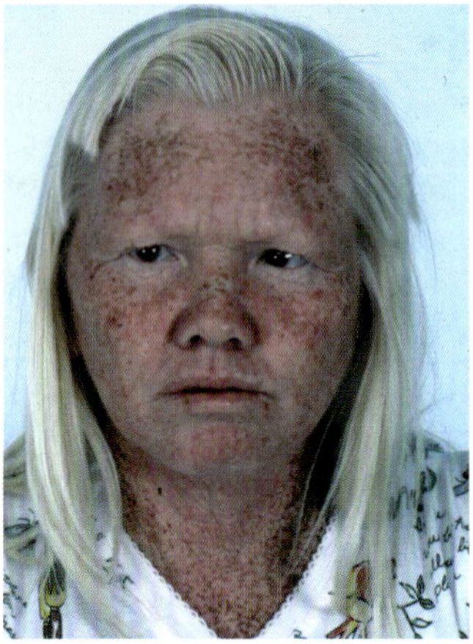

Oculocutaneous albinism and freckling in a Puerto Rican patient with Hermansky-Pudlak syndrome.

Age of onset

Birth

Epidemiology

High frequency in Puerto Rico, where 1:21 people are heterozygous carriers. Also, high frequency in a population isolate in the Swiss Alps.

Inheritance

Autosomal recessive

Chromosomal location

10q23 (HPS1); 15q11-q14 (AP3B1; HPS2); chromosomal location of the other Hermansky-Pudlak gene(s) is unknown.

Gene

The HPS1 gene is a novel gene of unknown function. AP3B1, mutated in HPS2, codes for the β-3A subunit of adaptin-3. The genes mutated in other forms of Hermansky-Pudlak syndrome are unknown.

Mutational spectrum

A 16 bp duplication in exon 15 of HPS1 accounts for the vast majority of Puerto Rican Hermansky-Pudlak patients, including all those from the northwest part of the Island. Other mutations in HPS1, including single base substitutions, insertions and deletions expected to result in premature truncation of the HPS1 protein, have been seen in Swiss, Irish, Japanese, Ukrainian and other ethnic groups. Only two brothers with AP3B1 mutations have been described to date. The causative gene(s) in patients whose HPS is not due to mutations in either HPS1 or AP3B1 has not yet been mapped or defined.

Effect of mutation

The Hermansky-Pudlak genes identified to date have mouse homologues that are known to cause pigment dilution and bleeding disorders in mice. The HPS1 gene is homologous to *pale ear*, and AP3B1 is homologous to mouse *pearl*. Mutations in these genes are expected to interfere with normal protein trafficking and vesicle formation from the trans-Golgi network to lysosomes, melanosomes and platelet dense bodies.

Diagnosis

Absence of platelet dense bodies on wet-mount electron microscopic examination confirms the clinical diagnosis for all types of Hermansky-Pudlak syndrome. The common 16 bp duplication in HPS1 can be diagnosed by a simple PCR-based test on genomic DNA. For HPS1 patients lacking the 16 bp duplication, SSCP followed by sequence analysis of exons showing abnormal migration patterns can identify the mutations.

Counselling issues

Death due to pulmonary fibrosis by the fourth or fifth decade is usual in patients with the 16 bp duplication, and also occurs in other HPS-1 patients. The frequency and severity of pulmonary fibrosis remains to be determined in other HPS patients.

Chediak-Higashi Syndrome

AKA

Chediak-Higashi-Steinbrinck disease; Beguez-Cesar-Chediak disease

MIM

214500

Clinical features

Decreased pigmentation of skin, hair and eyes, with a steel-grey or silvery appearance to the hair. Photophobia. Nystagmus. Neutropaenia. Increased susceptibility to common bacterial infections. Increased risk of unusual malignant lymphoma. Neurological involvement is variable.

Age of onset

Infancy to early childhood

Epidemiology

Very rare, with only 200 cases reported worldwide by the late 1980s

Inheritance

Autosomal recessive

Chromosomal location

1q42

Gene

LYST (sometimes called CHS1), a lysosomal trafficking regulator gene, of 11.4 kb, coding for a protein of 3801 amino acids.

Mutational spectrum

Premature stop codons produced by nonsense mutations or small deletions/insertions that predict a truncated protein.

Effect of mutation

The LYST gene is homologous to the mouse *beige* locus, making the *beige* phenotype an important animal model for Chediak-Higashi disease. The actual mechanism by which mutations in LYST cause clinical disease is unknown, although there is a suggestion that a defect in natural killer cell function may be involved.

Diagnosis

Large eosinophilic peroxidase-positive inclusion bodies (giant fused lysosomes) are seen in all cells with granules, including myeloblasts and pro-myelocytes in the bone marrow. Giant melanosomes are observed in melanocytes. It is possible that molecular diagnosis could be achieved by sequence analysis of the LYST gene from cDNA.

Counselling issues

Death usually occurs before age seven years, after a rapid downhill course of lymphoproliferation called the accelerated phase. Some atypical patients live to adulthood and show progressive neuropathy. It is possible that Chediak-Higashi disease is genetically heterogeneous, with loci other than LYST causing variants of the disease.

Piebaldism

AKA	White spot disease
MIM	172800
Clinical features	Depigmented, often symmetrical patches of skin with a predilection for the medial forehead, eyebrows, chin, chest, abdomen and limbs. The borders of the unpigmented areas are hyperpigmented. Most patients have a white forelock. Heterochromia irides. Epitheliomas.
Age of onset	Congenital
Epidemiology	Described in Japanese, African, middle Eastern and American Indian families among others
Inheritance	Autosomal dominant
Chromosomal location	4q11-q12
Gene	KIT, the human homologue of the v-kit Hardy-Zuckerman 4 feline sarcoma viral oncogene, which encodes 21 exons over 70 kb. Mutations in the mouse homologue of KIT cause dominant white spotting.
Mutational spectrum	Missense mutations and small deletions/insertions leading to premature truncation of the KIT protein
Effect of mutation	Interference with the tyrosine kinase receptor activity of the KIT protein may underly the clinical features of piebaldism.

Diagnosis

Combined SSCP and heteroduplex analysis of genomic DNA has been used to identify aberrant electrophoresis patterns, followed by sequence analysis to identify specific mutations.

Counselling issues

A high degree of intrafamilial variability. Hirschsprung disease and deafness have been reported in patients with piebaldism. Mutations in KIT, especially mutations occurring between codons 550 and 559, have been found in gastrointestinal stromal tumours. In addition, KIT mutations have been described in mastocytosis.

5

5. Disorders of Epidermal Appendages

Hypohidrotic/Anhidrotic Ectodermal Dysplasia

AKA Christ-Siemens-Touraine syndrome

MIM 305100

Clinical features Affected males have hypotrichosis, with fine, sparse and light-coloured scalp and body hair; however, beard hair is often normal. There is decreased to absent ability to sweat, which leads to heat intolerance. Hypodontia and conical or peg shaped teeth are usual. Facial features include periorbital hyperpigmentation, saddle nose and full lips. Defects in lacrimal and meibomian glands. Absent or accessory nipples in about 30%. Thick nasal secretions and cerumen.

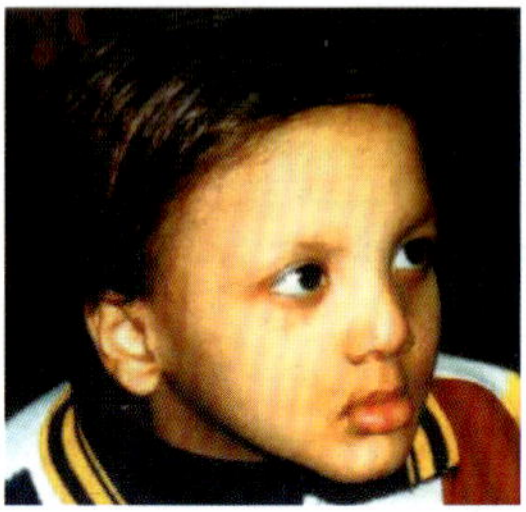

Typical facies of boy with hypohidrotic ectodermal dysplasia.

Age of onset Birth, with peeling skin and facial features often evident

Epidemiology Affects males (with variable findings in carrier females, due to random inactivation of the X chromosome that bears the normal gene). Most common of the ectodermal dysplasias. This disorder was first described by Darwin as "the toothless men of Sind", a large Hindu kindred. Seen in most ethnicities and races.

Inheritance X-linked recessive

Chromosomal location Xq12-q13.1

Gene

EDA, a gene with nine exons that encodes two alternative isoforms of a transmembrane protein

Mutational spectrum

Most mutations are missense, with a few nonsense or deletion mutations reported

Effect of mutation

The EDA locus in humans is homologous to the *tabby* locus in mice. EDA protein is expressed in hair follicles and adult epidermis, and EDA II isoform is proposed to play a role in tooth, hair and sweat gland morphogenesis.

Diagnosis

Both carrier females and affected males can be identified by direct genomic DNA sequence analysis or SSCP.

Counselling issues

Affected infants have increased risk of mortality, probably due to inability to regulate core temperature during episodes of fever. Carrier females often have mild clinical findings, including patchy areas of skin without sweating (mosaic hypohidrosis), missing or abnormally-shaped teeth and breast/nipple abnormalities. Due to lyonization of the X-chromosome, some females are severely affected.

Autosomal dominant and autosomal recessive forms of hypohidrotic ectodermal dysplasia are phenotypically indistinguishable from the X-linked form. The gene for these disorders maps to chromosome 2q (MIM 129490 and 224900, respectively), and they occur due to mutations in the human homologue of the mouse *downless* gene.

Ectodermal Dysplasia-Ectrodactyly-Cleft Lip/Palate Syndrome

AKA

EEC

MIM

129900 (EEC1); 602077 (EEC2); 604292 (EEC3)

Clinical features

Ectodermal dysplasia characterized by hypotrichosis with sparse, fine, dry scalp hair. Anodontia. Dystrophic and pitted nails. Less commonly hypohidrosis. Cleft lip and/or palate is present in some cases. Dysmorphic facies with facial short philtrum, broad nasal tip and maxillary hypoplasia is common. Ectrodactyly with split-hand/split-foot phenotype, or polysyndactyly without ectrodactyly. Ophthalmologic findings include blepharitis and keratitis. Dacryocystitis, probably secondary to tear duct anomalies, e.g. failure of canalization. Urinary tract and genital anomalies. Choanal atresia and lacrimal duct deformities.

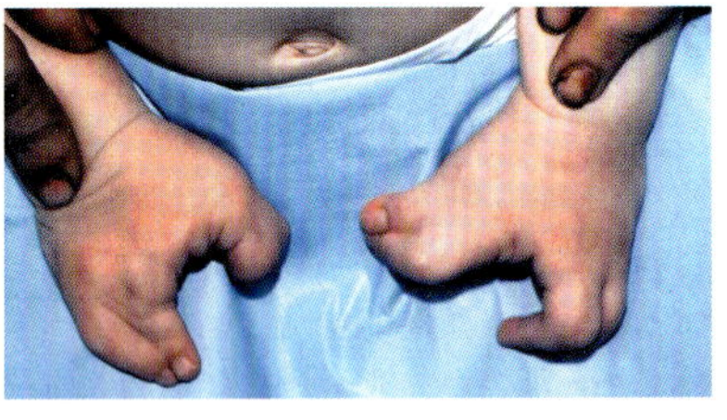

Split-hand deformity in EEC syndrome.
Photo courtesy of L.J. Russell, MD.

Age of onset

Congenital

Epidemiology

Reported in patients of many ethnic backgrounds, including Swedish, Belgian, English, Brazilian, Japanese, German and Dutch

Inheritance

Autosomal dominant

Chromosomal location

EEC1 (cytogenetic abnormality at 7q11.2-q21.3); EEC2 (chromosome 19); EEC3 (3q27)

Gene

The only gene identified in EEC is EEC3 on chromosome 3. Mutations in p63, which has strong homology to the p53 tumour-suppressor gene, have been identified. The underlying basis of the EEC types on chromosomes 7 and 19 are undefined.

Mutational spectrum

From a small series of patients in nine families, p63 mutations in EEC3 were observed resulting in $Arg^{204}Trp$, $Arg^{204}Gln$ and $Cys^{306}Arg$. A 1 bp insertion at nucleotide 1572 has been reported.

Effect of mutation

Mutations in the p63 gene are thought to abolish the DNA binding capacity of the resultant protein.

Diagnosis

Sequence analysis of genomic DNA

Counselling issues

Both intrafamilial and interfamilial variability make prediction of severity difficult. There is some suggestion that Rapp-Hodgkin type of ectodermal dysplasia (MIM 129400) is allelic to EEC, since individuals with a Rapp-Hodgkin diagnosis have been observed in pedigrees where other family members have the EEC phenotype. This is also true for lacrimoauriculodentodigital syndrome (MIM 149730).

Congenital Atrichia

AKA

Alopecia universalis congenita; atrichia congenita with papular lesions

MIM

203655; 209500

Clinical features

Congenital alopecia universalis. Some families have a variant phenotype with papular lesions over most of the body, but prominently on the knees and elbows.

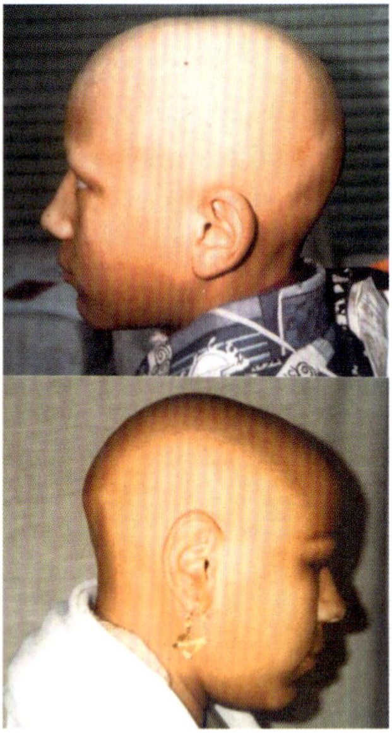

Congenital atrichia in brother and sister.

Age of onset

Hair is usually present at birth but falls out in the first weeks of life and never regrows.

Epidemiology

To date, described in inbred Pakistani, Arab and Irish Traveller families

Chromosomal location 8p21.2

Gene HR, the human homologue of the mouse *hairless* gene. HR is 14 kb long, and has 19 exons. It codes for a putative single zinc-finger transcription factor that is expressed in skin and brain.

Mutation spectrum Missense, splice-site and small deletion mutations leading to premature truncation of the HR protein. Deletion mutations are suggested to be associated with the papular phenotype while missense mutations may occur more often in families without the papular component of the disorder.

Effect of mutation HR mutations are hypothesised to impair the function of the zinc-finger domain in mediating binding of transcriptional co-activators to liganded nuclear receptors.

Diagnosis Can be accomplished by sequencing of either genomic or complementary DNA

Counselling issues In populations where the disease is frequent, and in families where it has been shown to occur, marriage between relatives carries a high risk of affected offspring.

Monilethrix

MIM

158000

Clinical features

Alopecia and broken hairs. Beaded hairs on light microscopic examination. Follicular plugging. There is variable expression; in some patients only hairs at the occiput are affected.

Age of onset

Before six months of age

Epidemiology

Most affected individuals are of European ancestry, but affected Asian Indian and Arab families have been described.

Inheritance

Autosomal dominant

Chromosomal location

12q13

Genes

HB1 or HB6; both hair keratin genes

Mutational spectrum

HB6 mutations causing $Glu^{413}Lys$ and $Glu^{413}Asp$ changes in the keratin protein have been described in several families. Also, $Asn^{114}His$ and $Asn^{114}Asp$ may occur. In the HB1gene, $Glu^{413}Lys$ and $Glu^{413}Lys$ have been observed.

Effect of mutation

Mutations are predicted to interfere with the assembly of keratin intermediate filaments. The abnormal filaments fail to give the hair normal strength and structure, and lead to fragility.

Diagnosis

Priority should be given to screening for the Glu^{413} mutations in both genes using restriction enzyme assays. Other mutations can be identified by direct sequencing of genomic DNA.

Counselling issues

Genetic heterogeneity is evident as there are reports of families that do not link to 12q13.

Tricho-Dento-Osseous Syndrome

AKA
TDO syndrome

MIM
190320

Clinical features
Hair is thick, coarse and kinky at birth, but may straighten over time. Nails may be thin and may peel. Small, pitted teeth with enamel hypoplasia. Taurodontism ("bull teeth"). Complete dental loss commonly occurs in early adulthood. Premature fusion of the cranial sutures results in dolichocephaly. There is increased density of the cranial bones.

Age of onset
Birth

Epidemiology
Several large US families have been described, and most can trace their ancestors back to the North Carolina, Virginia, Tennessee triangle area.

Inheritance
Autosomal dominant

Chromosomal location
17q12.3-q22

Gene
DLX3, a member of the distal-less homeobox gene family. The gene contains 3 exons. At least one other member of this gene family (DLX7) is 10 kb away.

Mutational spectrum
A common 4 bp deletion ^{3198}del4 has been described in many families, and there is evidence of a founder effect for the mutation.

Effect of mutation
Homeobox genes are expressed during embryonic development and are tissue and time specific in their expression pattern. In mice, defects in the DLX3 homologue have been shown to adversely affect development of the placenta, leading to early embryonic death of the pups.

Counselling issues

There can be considerable variation in clinical expression of the disease, despite the fact that the same mutation has been shown to cause most cases studied.

Tricho-Rhino-Phalangeal Syndromes

AKA
TRPSI; TRPSII (Langer-Giedion syndrome)

MIM
150230 (TRPS I); 190350 (TRPS II)

Clinical features
Features in common between the two tricho-rhino-phalangeal syndromes include sparse scalp hair, pear-shaped nose with bulbous tip, long philtrum and cone-shaped epiphyses. TRPS II is distinguished by redundant skin, bushy eyebrows, tented and thickened alae nasi, prune-belly, mental retardation, microcephaly and neonatal hypotonia. TRPS I patients are normocephalic and have normal intelligence.

Age of onset
Congenital

Epidemiology
All cases of TRPS II are sporadic, and most are male

Inheritance
TRPS I is autosomal dominant, while TRPS II is chromosomal (a contiguous gene syndrome).

Chromosomal location
Both syndromes map to 8q24; TRPS II has chromosomal deletions extending from 8q42.11 to 8q24.13

Gene
TRPS II is a contiguous gene syndrome, characterized by cytogenetically visible deletion of the end of the long arm of chromosome 8. TRPS I has mutations in a gene coding for a zinc-finger protein, thought to function as a transcription factor. The gene has been named TRPS1 and has seven exons.

Effect of mutation
Clinical features of TRPS type II are due to deletion of one copy of each of several genes on chromosome 8q, including EXT1 (a gene involved in cartilaginous exostoses) and TRPS1 (the gene mutated in TRPS type I). TRPS1 mutations are thought to cause clinical disease in TRPS I by inducing haplo-insufficiency.

Mutational spectrum

Six different mutations have been identified in ten unrelated patients. Three were nonsense mutations and three were insertional frameshift mutations. In all cases a truncated protein would be predicted.

Diagnosis

Cytogenetic analysis of an affected child with TRPS II will reveal terminal deletions of chromosome 8q. Cytogenetic analysis of parents of some affected children will identify balanced parental translocations that can increase the risk for recurrence in future offspring. For patients with TRPS I, genomic DNA is sequenced to identify mutations.

Counselling issues

There are similarities between TRPS I and II, but TRPS II is distinguished by neurological involvement including mental retardation. Dermatological differences include skin redundancy in TRPS II.

Nail-Patella Syndrome

AKA

Onychoosteodysplasia; Turner-Keiser syndrome; Fong disease; Oesterricher-Turner syndrome

MIM

161200

Clinical features

Triangular or V-shaped lunula. Nail dysplasia, usually symmetrical and ranging from mild to severe. Can include simple longitudinal ridging, clefting, splitting, abnormally-shaped or missing nails. Absent or hypoplastic patallae, subluxation/dislocation. Other features include iliac horns, elbow joint anomalies, abnormalities of scapulae and nephropathy.

Age of onset

Nail changes can be seen at birth; renal disease may also present in infancy

Epidemiology

Apparently not restricted to any particular population

Inheritance

Autosomal dominant

Chromosomal location

9q34.1

Gene

LMX1B, coding for a transcription factor of the LIM-homeodomain type, known to play a role in dorso-ventral patterning of the vertebrate limb.

Mutational spectrum

Many mutations in LMX1B result in premature termination of protein translation. $Arg^{200}Gln$ has been observed in several unrelated families. Most mutations affect exons 2 and 4; there are fewer in exons 3 and 5; and none have been reported in exons 1 and 6-8.

Effect of mutation

Most mutations affect the LIM and homeodomains and are hypothesised to cause loss of protein function. Loss of protein function from one allele suggests clinical disease is due to haplo-insufficiency of LMX1B protein.

Diagnosis

Sequencing of genomic DNA

Counselling issues

There is a founder effect reported in families of Italian ancestry. Sporadic cases of Nail-Patella syndrome due to new mutations are not uncommon.

Pachyonychia Congenita, Types I and II

AKA
PC1 Jadassohn-Lewandowsky type; PC2 Jackson-Lawler type

MIM
167200 (PC1); 167210 (PC2)

Clinical features
Thickened and friable finger and toe nails. Palm and sole hyperkeratosis and hyperhidrosis. Spiny follicular hyperkeratosis. PC2 patients may also have alopecia and natal teeth. PC1 patients often have oral leukoplakia, and this finding is absent in PC2.

Age of onset
Nail changes can usually be appreciated at birth

Inheritance
Autosomal dominant

Chromosomal location
17q12-q21; 12q13

Gene
Mutations have been found in two type I keratin genes, KRT17 (coding for keratin 17) and KRT16 (coding for keratin 16), on chromosome 17. Mutations have also been found in two type II keratin genes, KRT6B (coding for keratin 6b) and KRT6A (coding for keratin 6a), on chromosome 12.

Mutational spectrum
In PC2, KRT17 mutations resulting in $Asn^{92}Asp$, $Asn^{92}Ser$ and $Tyr^{98}Asp$, and mutations in KRT6B resulting in $Glu^{472}Lys$ have been described. In PC1, a mutation in KRT16 resulting in $Leu^{130}Pro$ and a 3 bp deletion in KRT6A at Asn^{8} have been described.

Effect of mutation
The presence of 50% abnormal keratin protein in the cell probably interferes with keratin intermediate filament stability.

Diagnosis
Direct sequencing of genomic DNA or cDNA. In large families, linkage studies may first identify the chromosomal locus to minimize the effort of screening four genes.

Counselling issues

Some reports suggest that PC may cause developmental delay.

Steatocystoma Multiplex

MIM	184500
Clinical features	Multiple (hundreds) of round or oval cysts (mm-cm size) presenting as dermal nodules of face, trunk, arms, back, thighs and scrotum. Cysts are filled with keratinaceous material and lipid, and occasionally small hairs. The cyst wall often contains sebaceous glands. Thickened nails. Leukonychia. Koilonychia.
Age of onset	Possibly congenital onset, but more likely childhood
Epidemiology	Rare
Inheritance	Autosomal dominant
Chromosomal location	17q12-q21
Gene	KRT17, coding for keratin 17, a type I (acidic) keratin located in the cluster of keratin genes on chromosome 17. The gene is 5 kb long with 8 exons and 7 introns and encodes a 432 amino acid protein expressed in nail bed, hair follicle, sebaceous glands and other epidermal appendages.
Mutational spectrum	Mutations resulting in $Arg^{94}His$ or $Arg^{94}Cys$ have been found in three families. Also seen is $Asn^{92}His$.
Effect of mutation	Mutations are expected to interfere with the stability of keratin intermediate filaments
Diagnosis	Direct sequence analysis of genomic DNA
Counselling issues	Malignant degeneration of a cyst in steatocystoma multiplex has been reported. KRT17 mutations have also been reported

in PC2, and there may be overlap in the clinical features between these disorders.

6. Disorders of the Dermis

Fabry Disease

AKA

Angiokeratoma corporis diffusum; α-galactosidase A deficiency; Anderson-Fabry disease

MIM

301500

Clinical features

Multiple angiokeratomas (vascular skin lesions), especially on the inner thighs and groin, with dark red-purple or black colour. Lesions can occur on oral mucosa. Hypohydrosis and heat intolerance. Lipid vascular fundus lesions and corneal dystrophy. Nephropathy leading to renal failure. Acute pain attacks. Autonomic dysfunction. Orthostatic hypotension. Thrombotic events. Cardiac involvement, including electrocardiogram (ECG) changes, angina and left ventricular wall and septal hypertrophy.

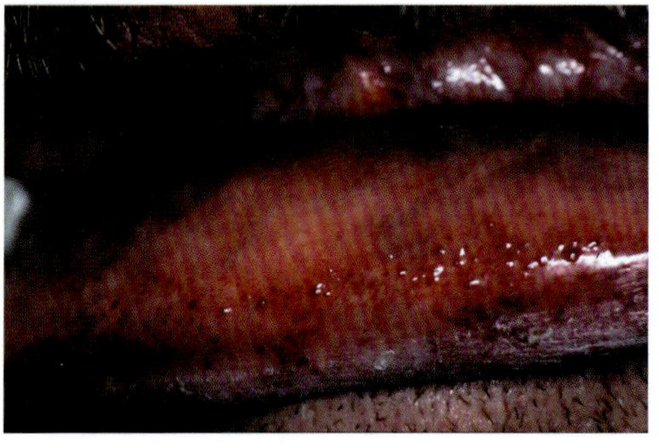

Multiple angiokeratomas of the lip in Fabry disease.
Photo courtesy of J.R. Toro, MD.

Age of onset

Mid-childhood

Epidemiology

Primarily affects males, but due to lyonization (X-inactivation) of the X-chromosome, heterozygous females can also be affected to some degree.

Inheritance

X-linked recessive

Chromosomal location	Xq22
Gene	GLA, coding for the α-galactosidase-A enzyme. The gene is 12 kb long and has 7 exons.
Mutational spectrum	Small deletions and missense mutations predominantly, with occasional nonsense mutations
Effect of mutation	Deficiency of α-galactosidase A results in lipid accumulation in various organs, particularly vascular tissue.
Laboratory findings	Maltese crosses (composed of crystalline glycosphingolipid) in urine under polarisation microscopy.
Diagnosis	Direct sequence analysis of genomic DNA
Counselling issues	Renal failure is a frequent cause of death, with the mean age of occurrence in the fifth decade of life.

Hereditary Haemorrhagic Telangiectasia

AKA	HHT; Osler-Weber-Rendu; Rendu-Osler-Weber
MIM	187300 (HHT1); 600376 (HHT2)
Clinical features	Telangiectasias, especially of mucosal surfaces (lips, tongue, nose and conjunctiva), palms, face, ears and fingers. Epistaxis. Telangiectasia of internal organs. Hypoxia and stroke. Brain abscesses. Bleeding from complication of pulmonary arteriovenous malformations. Bleeding from arteriovenous malformations at other anatomic sites is less common.
Age of onset	Epistaxis in childhood is usually the presenting feature. Systemic manifestations can also occur in childhood. Cutaneous manifestations present in teens or later. Penetrance is age-dependent, approaching 100% by age 40 years.
Epidemiology	Frequency estimated at 1:10,000-1:16,500
Inheritance	Autosomal dominant
Chromosomal location	9q33-q34.1; 12q11-q14
Gene	ENG (also known as CD105) is found on chromosome 9q and codes for endoglin, a homodimeric glycoprotein localized to the membrane of vascular endothelial cells. ACVRLK1, on chromosome 12q, codes for activin A receptor, type II-like kinase 1, a cell surface receptor for the TGF-β superfamily of ligands. The gene contains 9 exons, spanning over 15 kb. The protein, symbolised by ALK1, is found in endothelial cells and other highly vascularized tissue.
Mutational spectrum	ENG mutations appear to be private, with different mutations causing disease in different pedigrees. The mutations occur

throughout the gene and are primarily missense or splice-site. ACVRLK1 mutations include missense and small deletions.

Effect of mutation

Haplo-insufficiency for endoglin protein is thought to cause the clinical symptoms. Several mutations in ACVRLK1 resulting in null alleles suggest that haplo-insufficiency is also the mechanism for disease in these families.

Diagnosis

Linkage studies in appropriate families, followed by sequence analysis of genomic DNA

Counselling issues

It is important to distinguish HHT from other causes of epistaxis or telangiectasia. Pulmonary arteriovenous malformations appear to be more frequent in families with linkage to chromosome 9 and mutations in ENG, while they appear to be absent in non-chromosome 9 linked families with HHT.

Autosomal dominant hereditary benign telangiectasia (MIM 187260) does not involve systemic problems seen in HHT. All families with multiple telangiectasia should be evaluated for HHT.

Hereditary Angiooedema

AKA
Hereditary angioneurotic oedema; HANE

Inheritance
Autosomal dominant

Clinical features
Recurrent angiooedema with swelling of subcutaneous tissue and mucosa. Episodes of non-pruritic, non-urticarial, non-pitting oedema. A major complication is laryngeal oedema. Visceral oedema leading to gastrointestinal symptoms, including abdominal pain, nausea, vomiting and diarrhoea.

Age of onset
Usually begins in the toddler years

Epidemiology
Clinical features are more frequent in women than men (M:F ratio=0.85)

Chromosomal location
11q11-q13

Mutated gene
C1NH, coding for C1-esterase inhibitor. The gene has 8 exons.

Mutational spectrum
Splice-site and promoter sequence mutations, as well as missense and nonsense mutations

Effect of mutation
Mutations result in deficiency or decreased function of C1-esterase inhibitor, type I. The normal function of C1-esterase inhibitor is to regulate the first component of complement by inhibiting the proteolytic activity of two of its subcomponents.

Diagnosis
Mutation screening has been performed by fluorescence-assisted mismatch analysis or PCR and sequence analysis of genomic DNA.

Counselling issues
Type I hereditary angiooedema, where levels of C1NH are greatly reduced, accounts for 85% of the cases. In type II hereditary

angiooedema, clinically-indistinguishable from type I, serum levels are normal.

Polycystic ovaries are seen with increased frequency in patients with hereditary angiooedema. Homozygosity for a promoter mutation, implying autosomal recessive inheritance, has been described in one family.

Ehlers-Danlos Syndrome, Classical Type

AKA Ehlers-Danlos syndrome, Gravis (type I); Ehlers-Danlos syndrome, Mitis (type II)

MIM 130000; 130010

Clinical features Similar cutaneous features are shared by the Gravis and Mitis types, with the mitis type being milder. Fragile skin. Easy bruising. Cigarette-paper scarring. Lax and velvety skin texture. Systemic features include joint and ligament laxity with dislocation, mitral valve prolapse, hiatus hernia, bowel and bladder diverticula, bowel and arterial rupture and retinal detachment.

Age of onset Prenatal with premature rupture of membranes and premature birth

Epidemiology Seen in many ethnic groups

Inheritance Autosomal dominant

Chromosomal location 2q31; 9q34.2-34.3

Genes COL5A1, on chromosome 9, coding for the α-1 chain of type 5 collagen, and COL5A2, on chromosome 2, coding for the α-2 chain. Type 5 collagen occurs as a heterotrimer of α-1, α-2 and α-3 chains, or two α-1 chains and one α-2 chain, or as an α-1 homotrimer. It is expressed in placenta and skin (and as a minor collagen component in many other tissues), and is suggested to have important functions in development and wound healing. COL5A1 has 66 exons over 750 kb; other collagen genes have 52.

Mutational spectrum Splice site mutations leading to in-frame exon skipping, point mutations primarily affecting cysteine residues and other missense mutations have been identified in both COL5A1 and COL5A2.

Effect of mutation

Mutated collagen chains are incapable of being incorporated into collagen trimers

Diagnosis

Abnormal electrophoretic activity of pro-α-1 or pro-α-2 chains can be detected in collagen type 5 obtained from cultured fibroblast cells from some, but not all, affected individuals. CSGE of genomic DNA, followed by sequence analysis of exons with abnormal patterns, and heteroduplex analysis have been used to identify mutations in the very large collagen genes.

Counselling issues

Children with Ehlers-Danlos syndrome, Classical type, have mistakenly been thought to be victims of child abuse due to the presence of bruises and poorly healing wounds from minor trauma.

Ehlers-Danlos Syndrome, Vascular Type

AKA

Ehlers-Danlos, Arterial type; Ehlers-Danlos, Ecchymotic type; Ehlers-Danlos, Sack-Barabas type; Ehlers-Danlos type IV

MIM

130050

Clinical features

Fragile, thin, translucent skin with easy bruising. Atrophic and premature-aged appearance of skin over acral areas (fingers, nose and ears). Prominent venous markings. Mild skin hyperextensibility. Joint hypermobility limited to fingers. Acrogeric appearance of face, with pinched nose and thin lips. Acro-osteolysis of feet and hands.

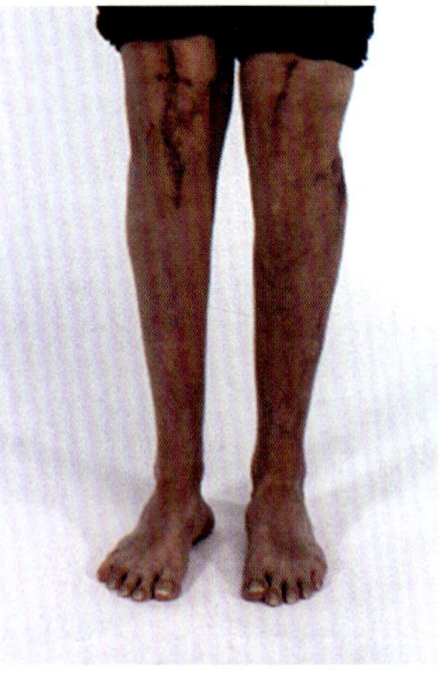

Scars in a young woman with Ehlers-Danlos Syndrome, Vascular type resulting from surgical repair of patellar and quadriceps tendon ruptures occurring in her teens. The patient also had a uterine tear with her first pregnancy.
Photo courtesy of G. Hostetter, M.D.

Age of onset

Infancy to late teens or early adulthood

Inheritance

Autosomal dominant

Chromosomal location

2q31

Gene

COL3A1, coding for the α-1 chain of collagen 3. Type III collagen is expressed in foetal tissue and adult blood vessels.

Mutational spectrum

There are about 25 reported mutations, half of which affect glycine residues (with a change to another amino acid) and the remainder causing skipping of exons in the protein translation. A $Gly^{571}Ser$ mutation in one large family seemed to incur a milder phenotype.

Effect of mutation

Mutations result in a deficiency of type III collagen in dermal fibroblasts due to defective synthesis. Since three chains of pro-α-1 collagen are required to form type III pro-collagen, a mutation in one allele of COL3A1 results in only half-normal numbers of α-1 chains. This leads to assembly of only 1/8 normal pro-collagen III molecules and 7/8 abnormal pro-collagen III molecules.

Diagnosis

DGGE of PCR-amplified cDNA from the C-terminal domain of the type III collagen can be used to identify mutations in the large COL3A1 gene.

Counselling issues

Risk of death to women during pregnancy is very high (25% in one series) due to rupture of bowel, aorta, vena cava or uterus, laceration of the vaginal wall during delivery or postpartum haemorrhage. Death usually occurs by age 40 due to bowel rupture or rupture of major blood vessels. There is some suggestion that a recessive form of Ehlers-Danlos syndrome, vascular type may exist.

Ehlers-Danlos Syndrome, Arthrochalasia Type

AKA

Arthrochalasia multiplex congenita; Ehlers-Danlos type 7A (EDS 7A); Ehlers-Danlos type 7B (EDS 7B)

MIM

130060

Clinical features

Hyperextensible and bruisable skin. Short stature. Small mandible. Flaccid joints. Fractures are seen in some Ehlers-Danlos syndrome, Kyphoscoliosis type patients.

Age of onset

Birth

Inheritance

Autosomal dominant

Chromosomal location

17q21.31-q22.05 (EDS 7A); 7q22.1 (EDS 7B)

Mutated gene

COL1A1 (52 exons), on chromosome 17, in EDS 7A, and COL1A2 (51 exons) on chromosome 7, in EDS 7B

Mutational spectrum

Most families have distinct mutations altering the consensus splice junction of exon 6 in COL1A1 or COL1A2. These result in exon 6 being spliced out of the message and also cause in-frame deletions of 24 or 18 amino acid residues in the pro-α-1 (I) or pro-α-2 (I) chains, respectively.

Effect of mutation

Mutations alter the protease cleavage site in either the pro-α-1 or pro-α-2 chains of type I collagen. The COL1A1 mutations produce more severe phenotypic effects than COL1A2 mutations, probably because heterotrimeric collagen I consists of two α-1 chains, but only one α-2 chain. Alterations in mineral deposition on collagen fibrils in bony tissue lead to increased risk of fracture.

Diagnosis

The COL1A1 and COL1A2 mutations which result in deletions can be identified by screening cDNA.

Counselling issues

COL1A1 and COL1A2 mutations are very frequently associated with osteogenesis imperfecta types II and III, with most mutations being missense changes affecting glycine residues.

Ehlers-Danlos Syndrome Dermatosparaxis Type

AKA Ehlers-Danlos syndrome type VII C

MIM 225410

Inheritance Autosomal recessive

Clinical features Soft, velvety, doughy and elastic skin that is extremely fragile and tears with little trauma. Facial appearance is striking, with epicanthal folds, depressed nasal bridge, small chin, large-appearing eyes with blue sclerae and thickened eyelids. Umbilical hernia. Short stature.

Age of onset Congenital. Premature rupture of membranes and premature birth have been reported in several children.

Epidemiology Rare. The biochemical and genetic basis of the disease was first identified in cattle; it also occurs in Himalayan cats and sheep.

Chromosomal location Unknown

Gene ADAMTS2 (aka hPCPNI), coding for pro-collagen I N-proteinase, the enzyme that excises the N-propeptide of type I and type II pro-collagens

Mutational spectrum Most patients (5/6) are homozygous for a mutation resulting in Glu^{225}Stop, which terminates protein translation prematurely. One patient was homozygous for a different truncating mutation, Trp^{795}Stop.

Effect of mutation Mutations result in deficiency of pro-collagen I N-proteinase

Diagnosis

Assay of pro-collagen processing in cultured fibroblasts and direct DNA sequence analysis of PCR-fragments to detect the two reported mutations.

Counselling issues

Inguinal tears are reported to occur at birth. Suturing of the skin in patients with dermatosparaxis is very difficult due to its extreme fragility.

X-linked Cutis Laxa

AKA Occipital horn syndrome; Ehlers-Danlos syndrome type IX

MIM 304150

Clinical features Droopy, loose, lax skin (cutis laxa). Velvety skin with somewhat easy bruisability. Hypermobile and lax joints. Bony prominences on each side of the foramen magnum. Bladder and GI diverticuli. Chronic diarrhoea. Hernias of the diaphragm, abdomenal wall and inguinal canals. Generalized skeletal dysplasia including broad clavicles and pectus abnormalities. Mild mental retardation is common.

Age of onset Birth

Epidemiology Restricted to males

Inheritance X-linked recessive

Chromosomal location Xq12-q13

Mutated gene ATP7A, coding for a Cu^{2+}-transporting ATPase, α-peptide. The gene contains 23 exons in 150 kb of DNA and displays striking homology to the gene causing Wilson disease (ATP7B), an autosomal recessive disorder of copper metabolism.

Mutational spectrum Several deletion mutations are described that lead to exon skipping, particularly involving exon 8. Mutations in ATP7A are also responsible for Menkes kinky hair syndrome (see page 168).

Effect of mutation Lack of Cu^{2+}-transporting ATPase activity leads to defects in copper uptake and abnormality of other copper-dependent enzyme activity and protein cross-links.

Diagnosis

Decreased serum copper and ceruloplasmin levels can be identified. Carrier DNA sequencing should reveal the deletion mutations, but genomic DNA sequencing may be needed to identify the rarer missense mutations.

Counselling issues

The name, cutis laxa, is applied to a group of disorders characterized by lax skin. There are autosomal dominant and recessive forms of the disease, as well as the X-linked form. Only the X-linked form has been reported to have occipital horns.

7. Other Hereditary Disorders with Skin Manifestations

Leprechaunism

AKA Donohue syndrome

MIM 246200

Clinical features Hirsutism. Pachyderma (redundancy of skin). Loss of subcutaneous tissue. Wrinkling. Elfin facies with thick lips. Large genitalia. Umbilical and inguinal hernia. Myocardial hypertrophy. Prenatal growth retardation. Microcephaly.

Age of onset Prenatal

Epidemiology Parents are often consanguineous

Inheritance Autosomal recessive

Chromosomal location 19p13.2

Gene INSR, coding for the insulin receptor, a tetramer of two α- and two β-subunits. The gene is 120 kb long and contains 22 exons. It codes for a 1370 amino acid protein.

Mutational spectrum A variety of missense mutations have been reported

Effect of mutation Resistance to insulin leading to severe hyperinsulinaemia, fasting hypoglycaemia and post-prandial hyperglycaemia. Mutations in INSR may also affect the epidermal growth factor receptor.

Diagnosis Molecular diagnosis by DNA sequence analysis. Prenatal diagnosis in families at risk is possible if the mutation is known, or by evaluation of insulin receptor function in cultured amniocytes.

Counselling issues

Affected children usually die in infancy. Mutations in INSR have also been found in some individuals with insulin-resistant diabetes mellitus.

Menkes Syndrome

AKA	Kinky hair disease
MIM	309400
Clinical features	Sparse hair, eyebrows and lashes at birth. Hair is fine, kinky, silver-steel in colour and the shafts break easily. Skin is lax, with cutis marmorata pattern. Hypothermia, spasticity and seizures in infancy. Growth failure and developmental delay.
Age of onset	Infancy
Epidemiology	Affects males, with an estimated frequency of 1:40,000 births in Melbourne, Australia and 1:298,000 births in Europe
Inheritance	X-linked recessive
Chromosomal location	Xq12-q13
Gene	ATP7A, coding for a Cu^{2+}-transporting ATPase, α-peptide. The gene contains 23 exons in 150 kb of DNA, and has striking homology to the gene causing Wilson disease (ATP7B), an autosomal recessive disorder of copper metabolism.
Mutational spectrum	Most mutations result in a truncated protein product. Mutations in ATP7A are also responsible for X-linked cutis laxa.
Effect of mutation	Abnormal copper transport across membranes results in global copper deficiency. Copper-dependent enzymes are active in many systems, including mitochondria, hair, skin, skeleton and brain (synthesis of neurotransmitters).
Diagnosis	Elevated serum ceruloplasmin levels. Direct DNA diagnosis can be accomplished by genomic DNA sequence analysis.

Counselling issues

Death usually occurs in the first year of life. Neurologically normal carrier females may have some hairs that show pili torti and some uneven skin pigmentation. Some affected males with milder phenotypes have been reported to survive into the teen years.

Variegate Porphyria

MIM

176200

Clinical features

Photosensitivity leading to blistering, then milia, hyperpigmentation and hypertrichosis. Acute neuro-visceral attacks, which can be induced by exposure to drugs.

Age of onset

Early adult life

Epidemiology

Common in South Africans of Dutch descent, otherwise it is rare. Some have suggested that King George III of England had variegate porphyria.

Inheritance

Autosomal dominant

Chromosomal location

1q22-q23

Gene

PPOX, coding for protoporphyrinogen oxidase. The gene is 5 kb in length, and has 1 non-coding and 12 coding exons.

Mutational spectrum

The majority of affected South Africans (80%) have a mutation leading to $Arg^{59}Trp$ in the protein. In Europeans, a variety of missense, frame-shift, splice site and nonsense mutations have been described.

Effect of mutation

Mutations in the enzyme lead to the inability to convert protoporphyrinogen IX to protoporphyrin IX in the pathway of haem biosynthesis.

Diagnosis

Blood, urine and stool screening for porphyrin excretion.
A pattern of porphobilinogen in blood, porphobilinogen and δ-aminolevulinic acid in urine (during attacks), and increased proto-and coproporphyrin in stool is consistent with the diagnosis.

Direct sequencing of the PPOX gene from genomic DNA confirms the diagnosis.

Counselling issues

A mutation in the HFE gene, responsible for hereditary haemochromatosis in many patients, has also been found in a patient with porphyria. Detection of asymptomatic patients is important so they can be advised to avoid exposure to agents that provoke neuro-visceral attacks.

Congenital Erythropoetic Porphyria

AKA Gunther disease

MIM 263700

Clinical features Photosensitivity leading to blistering and scarring. Hypertrichosis and hyperpigmentation. Haemolytic anaemia. Thrombocytopaenia. Bleeding diathesis. Jaundice. Hepatosplenomegaly. Growth and developmental delay. Pink-reddish teeth. Pink urine.

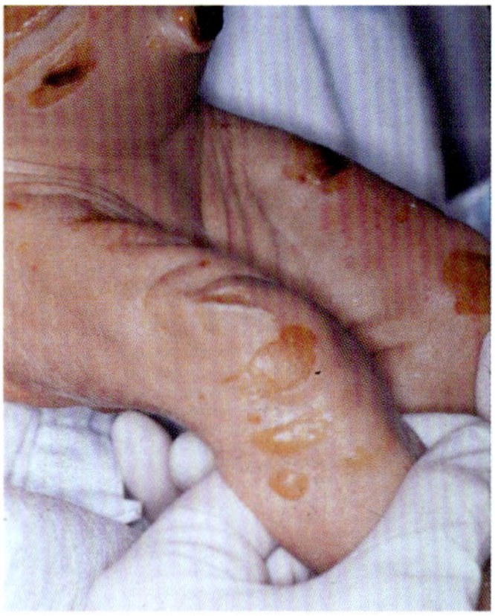

Multiple vescicle and bullae in infant with congential erythropoetic porphyria. Photo courtesy of J.R. Toro, MD.

Age of onset Variable, from birth to adulthood

Epidemiology Very rare

Inheritance Autosomal recessive

Chromosomal location 10q25.2-q26.3

Gene UROIIIS, coding for the enzyme uroporphyrinogen III synthase (UROS). The gene has 10 exons.

Mutational spectrum

Variety of missense, nonsense, frameshift and splicing mutations. $Cys^{73}Arg$ is reported to be more frequent than other mutations and accounts for some 40% of UROIIIS disease alleles.

Effect of mutation

Mutations lead to defects in the activity of the uroporphyrinogen III synthase enzyme in the haem biosynthesis pathway.

Diagnosis

Exposure of teeth and diaper to Wood's lamp shows fluorescent red colouring. Increased copro-, uro- and protoporphyrin in blood, and increased uro- and coproporphyrin in urine and faeces are consistent with the diagnosis. Direct genomic DNA analysis will reveal UROIIIS mutations and can be used for prenatal diagnosis.

Counselling issues

Death usually ensues by the fifth decade. Heterozygotes for a mutation in UROIIIS may be detectable due to their intermediate levels of UROS enzyme activity.

Porphyria Cutanea Tarda (PCT) and Hepatoerythropoietic Porphyria (HEP)

AKA

Type II porphyria cutanea tarda; familial porphyria cutanea tarda

MIM

176100

Clinical features

Light-sensitive dermatosis characterized by bullae and vesicles that heal with scarring. Skin is fragile to trauma. Hyperpigmentation. Hypertrichosis. Hepatic involvement (including chronic renal failure, cirrhosis and/or hepatoma).

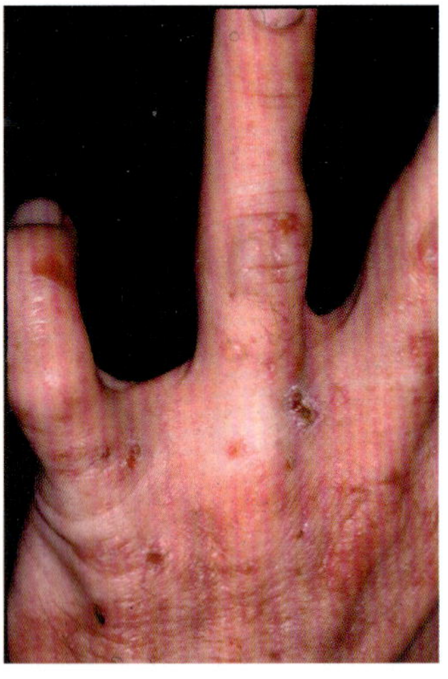

Vescicles and erosions on the dorsum of the hand in porphyria cutanea tarda.
Photo courtesy of J.R. Toro, MD

Age of onset

Light-sensitive episodes, which can be exacerbated by alcohol or oestrogen use, occur in adults with PCT. Homozygotes with HEP present with skin findings in infancy.

Epidemiology

PCT is more common in men than women and occurs worldwide, with a particularly high frequency in the Bantu of South Africa. The homozygous state, represented by HEP, is very rare.

Inheritance

PCT is autosomal dominant; HEP is the homozygous state (two copies of the mutated dominant gene)

Chromosomal location

1p34

Gene

UROD, coding for the enzyme uroporphyrinogen decarboxylase, the fifth enzyme of the haem biosynthetic pathway. The gene has 10 exons over 3 kb.

Mutational spectrum

Gly^{281}Val causes PCT, while homozygous Gly^{281}Glu is found in HEP. Other splice mutations are found in both PCT and HEP which lead to deletion of a complete exon, and missense mutations are described in PCT.

Effect of mutation

Mutations result in deficiency of uroporphyrinogen decarboxylase. Heterozygotes have 50% of normal levels of the enzyme, while homozygotes with HEP have less than 10% of normal levels in red cells and cultured fibroblasts.

Diagnosis

Laboratory findings include increased iron storage in all tissues, increased uroporphyrin and iso-coproporphyrin in urine, and increased iso-coproporphyrin (and other porphyrins) in faeces. Sequence analysis of the UROD gene from genomic DNA confirms the diagnosis and can be used for counselling purposes.

Counselling issues

Many cases of PCT are sporadic and many heterozygotes remain symptom-free until challenged by environmental factors. There is some evidence that mutations in HFE (the gene involved in haemochromatosis) contribute to disease expression in PCT.

Cerebrotendinous Xanthomatosis

AKA	Cerebral cholesterinosis; cholestanolosis
MIM	213700
Clinical features	Xanthalasma (thick yellow or flesh-coloured nodules and plaques) representing large deposits of cholesterol and cholestanol. Every tissue may be involved, especially Achilles tendon, brain and lungs. Progressive neurodegeneration. Premature atherosclerosis. Cataracts.
Age of onset	Usually by second decade of life, but neurological impairment may appear later
Epidemiology	Rare. The gene frequency is estimated at 1:108 in Moroccan Sephardic Jews. The disease has also been reported in the Netherlands and Japan, and in black individuals.
Inheritance	Autosomal recessive
Chromosomal location	2q33-qter
Gene	CYP27, encoding sterol 27-hydroxylase, a mitochondrial cytochrome P450 enzyme important in the bile acid biosynthesis pathway. The gene has 9 exons over 18.6 kb.
Mutational spectrum	Mostly missense mutations affecting arginine residues. Moroccan Jews are reported to have either a 16 bp deletion in exon 4 or an intron 4 splice acceptor site mutation.
Effect of mutation	Decreased activity of the CYP27 enzyme leads to build up of cholestanol which is deposited in tissues.

Diagnosis

Patients have normal plasma cholesterol levels, while cholestanol is present in abnormal amounts in serum and tendon tissue. Molecular diagnosis can be accomplished by sequencing of genomic DNA.

Counselling issues

Treatment with chenodeoxycholic acid (CDCA) results in clinical improvement.

Wiskott-Aldrich Syndrome

AKA Aldrich syndrome

MIM 301000

Clinical features Eczema, with secondary infection common. Thrombocytopaenia with petechiae and purpura. Bloody diarrhoea.
Unusual susceptibility to bacterial and viral infection.

Age of onset Early childhood

Epidemiology The original descriptions were of patients with Dutch and German ancestry. In the United States, the frequency has been estimated at 1:250,000 male births.

Inheritance X-linked recessive

Chromosomal location Xp11.23-p11.22

Gene WAS, spanning about 9 kb and containing 12 exons. The WAS protein has a GTPase binding site and is expressed only in lymphocytic and megakaryocytic cell lineages.

Mutational spectrum About half the mutations result in premature truncation of WAS protein translation. Most of the mutations are unique to each family, although Arg^{86} missense mutations have been reported in several patients. Exons 1 and 2 may have mutational hotspots.

Effect of mutation The immune defect in Wiskott-Aldrich syndrome is one of antigen processing or recognition. The WAS protein may regulate organization of the actin cytoskeleton, a structure that is severely disturbed in T lymphocytes of affected males.

Diagnosis

SSCP followed by sequencing of exons showing aberrant electrophoretic patterns

Counselling issues

Death usually occurs before 10 years of age due to infection, bleeding or malignancy. Bone marrow transplantation has been used to treat Wiskott-Aldrich syndrome. There have been suggestions that both autosomal dominant and autosomal recessive forms of the disease exist. Mutations in WAS have also been found in X-linked congenital thrombocytopaenia, a disorder with no abnormalities of lymphoid cells.

Chronic Granulomatous Disease

MIM

306400; 233690; 233700; 233710

Clinical features

Recurrent skin infections. Pyodermas with regional lymphadenopathy. Periorificial dermatitis. Perianal staphylococcal abscesses. Cutaneous granulomas. Intraoral and perioral ulcers. Gingivitis. Scalp folliculitis. Severe seborrhoeic dermatitis. Suppurative lymphadenitis. Hepatosplenomegaly and hepatic granuloma. Pneumonia. Carrier females (for the X-linked type) do not have an increased risk of infection, but may have systemic lupus erythematosis-like skin changes.

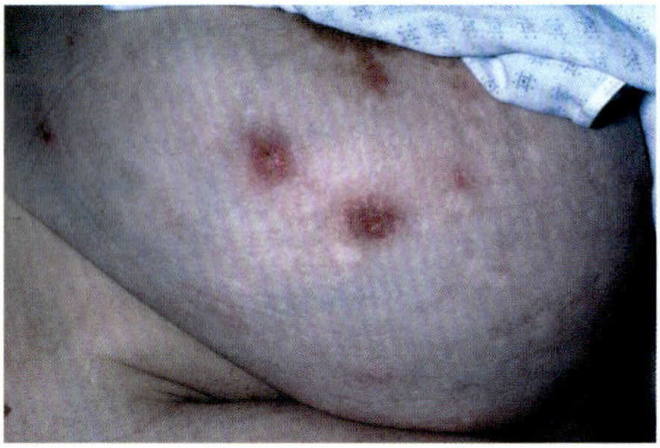

Cutaneous granulomas in chronic granulomatous disease. Photo courtesy of J.R. Toro, MD.

Age of onset

Within the first year of life

Epidemiology

Mutations in boys affected with the X-linked type of chronic granulomatous disease are nearly always inherited from carrier mothers (i.e. they are not due to new mutations). However, the proportion of sporadic carrier females (women who inherited a new CYBB gene mutation from an unaffected father) is high, suggesting that most new mutations in CYBB arise in male gametes.

Inheritance

X-linked recessive (MIM 306400); autosomal recessive (233690, 233700, 233710)

Chromosomal location

Xp21.1 (the X-linked type); 1q25 (autosomal recessive; NCF2), 16q24 (autosomal recessive; CYBA) and 7q11 (autosomal recessive; NCF1).

Gene

CYBB, coding for the 91 kDa glycoprotein component (p91-*phox*) of NADPH oxidase. The gene encompasses 13 exons spanning approximately 30 kb of DNA. The three autosomal recessive genes are: NCF2, coding for the p67*phox* component; CYBA, coding for the p22*phox* component; and NCF1, coding for the p47*phox* component.

Mutational spectrum (CYBB)

Most mutations are private, occurring independently in each family. In a large series of X-linked chronic granulomatous disease patients the following mutations were observed: large and small deletions (11%); frame-shift mutations (24%); nonsense mutations (23%); missense mutations (23%); splice region mutations (17%); and regulatory region mutations (2%).

Effect of mutation

The mutations render the NADPH oxidase system unable to perform its normal function of producing superoxide and other toxic oxygen metabolites. Thus, although leukocytes are able to phagocytose bacteria, they are not able to digest and kill them.

Diagnosis

SSCP screening followed by sequence analysis of exons showing abnormal migration patterns on electrophoresis

Counselling issues

The existence of both X-linked and autosomal recessive forms of the disease makes it very important to get an accurate family history from patients. It is most likely that an affected male has the X-linked form, since it accounts for 65-80% of chronic granulomatous disease. The diagnosis of the full disorder in a female child strongly suggests the recessive form. In the X-linked form of the disease, cytochrome b_{558} is not detectable at all, while most patients with a recessive form have normal cytochrome b_{558} levels. Bone marrow transplant has been an effective treatment in some patients.

Hereditary Lymphoedema Type I

AKA

Primary congenital lymphoedema; Nonne-Milroy lymphoedema; Milroy disease

MIM

153100

Clinical features

Bilateral oedema of the lower extremities (often congenital), and sometimes the upper extremities. Scrotal swelling.

Age of onset

Prenatal (diagnosed by ultrasound) to mid-50s. Penetrance is estimated at 80%.

Epidemiology

Most published families are Western European, North American or British. A male:female ratio of 1:2.3 has been reported.

Inheritance

Autosomal dominant

Chromosomal location

5q35.3

Gene

FLT4, coding for the vascular endothelial growth factor C receptor. FLT4 mRNA is expressed in lymphatic endothelia and some high endothelial venules.

Mutational spectrum

In a single family, the missense mutation $Pro^{1126}Leu$ has been identified

Effect of mutation

It is hypothesized that abnormal vascular endothelial growth factor receptor impairs vasculogenesis.

Diagnosis

Sequence analysis of complementary DNA

Counselling issues

There is an increased risk of infection in involved extremities and also a risk of developing angiosarcoma in long-standing lymphoedema. Other hereditary lymphoedemas (e.g. lymphoedema praecox and lymphoedema with distichiasis) have not yet been mapped to a chromosomal location.

Cockayne Syndrome (CS)

AKA

Cockayne syndrome A (CSA); Cockayne syndrome B (CSB) based on complementation studies.

MIM

216400

Clinical features

Sun sensitivity with skin atrophy but without the pigmentary changes or skin cancers found in xeroderma pigmentosum (XP). Dwarfism. Precocious senile (Progeria-like) appearance. Optic atrophy. Deafness. Progressive neurological degeneration, mental retardation and dementia. Gait abnormalities.

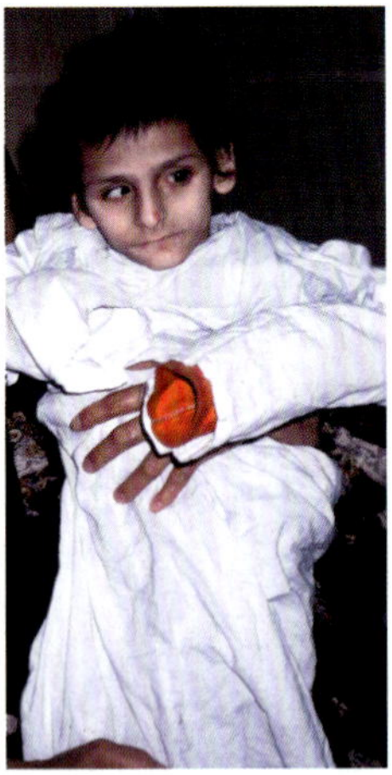

13 year old boy with Cockayne syndrome.

Laboratory features

CS cells are abnormally sensitive to ultraviolet radiation and are defective in the repair of transcriptionally active genes.

Age of onset

Early childhood

Epidemiology

Rare. The disorder can also be seen in association with XP (see page 38) in the xeroderma pigmentosum/Cockayne syndrome phenotype.

Inheritance

Autosomal recessive

Chromosomal location

Chromosome 5 (CSA); 10q11 (CSB)

Genes

Mutations in two genes have been described in CS without XP. In CSA, the CKN1 gene, is predicted to produce a WD repeat (WD-40 repeat) protein, a highly conserved sequence of repeating units usually ending with Trp-Asp. In CSB, mutations in ERCC6 have been identified. In addition, the xeroderma pigmentosum/Cockayne syndrome phenotype may be associated with mutations in the XPB, XPD or XPG genes.

Mutational spectrum

Large deletions and nonsense mutations resulting in a truncated protein or protein with internal deletions have been found in CKN1. Nonsense mutations and small deletions/insertions have been described in ERCC6.

Effect of mutation

Mutations in the genes associated with CS appear to cause defects in RNA polymerase II-mediated RNA transcription.

Diagnosis

Hypersensitivity of fibroblasts to killing by UV or delayed recovery of RNA synthesis after exposure of cells to UV. Mutation identification can be accomplished by sequence analysis of genomic or complementary DNA.

Counselling issues

Death ensues at an early age due to general cachexia or atherosclerosis. The relationship between CS and XP is still unclear.

Werner Syndrome

AKA Progeria of the adult

MIM 277700

Clinical features Scleroderma-like skin changes with loss of subcutaneous tissue and epidermal and dermal atrophy. Thinning and greying of hair. Balding. Subcutaneous calcification. Patchy hypo- and hyperpigmentation. Cataract. Prematurely aged and wizened facies. Arteriosclerosis. Diabetes mellitus. Short stature due to growth arrest at puberty. Hypogonadism. Slender limbs and stocky trunk. Beaked nose. High-pitched voice.

Age of onset Premature aging develops in the second to third decade of life

Epidemiology Three per million in Japan. Estimates of carrier frequency are as high as 1:150-1:200.

Inheritance Autosomal recessive

Chromosomal location 8p12-p11.2

Gene WRN, coding for a predicted 1432 amino acid protein with homology to DNA and RNA helicases (unwinding proteins). The gene has 35 exons, with the coding sequence beginning in exon 2.

Mutational spectrum A single splice-site mutation (IV525DS, G-C, -1) resulting in a frame-shift and a truncated protein is found to be homozygous in 60% of Japanese patients. There are a variety of mutations in patients of other ethnic backgrounds, and virtually all predict premature termination of protein translation.

Effect of mutation

The mutations predict complete loss of function of the WRN product. Werner syndrome fibroblasts and immortalized B-lymphocytes are sensitive to some DNA-damaging agents. Cells from Werner syndrome patients also show an increased rate of chromosome aberration. It is thought that the WRN gene product is involved in some aspect of DNA replication, possibly unwinding of DNA strands, or in telomere formation or function.

Diagnosis

An allele-specific PCR-based assay is used to screen for common mutations. Sequencing of cDNA prepared from mRNA isolated from lymphoblastoid lines or direct sequence analysis of genomic DNA is used to identify the less common mutations.

Counselling issues

The mean age of death is in the 40s, frequently due to atherosclerosis or a variety of non-cutaneous malignancies. Glaucoma also occurs frequently in Werner syndrome patients.

Conradi-Hunermann Syndrome

AKA Chondrodysplasia punctata; Happle syndrome

MIM 302960

Clinical features Cicatricial scarring. Alopecia. Ichthyosis which may be patchy or diffuse and when faded leaves linear or whorled atrophoderma and pigmentation, sometimes along the lines of Blaschko. Aberrant punctate calcification in epiphyseal cartilage. Asymmetric rhizomelic limb shortening. Cataracts. Deafness.

Age of onset Congenital, sometimes with the remnants of a collodion membrane visible. The punctate calcifications and ichthyotic changes usually resolve during infancy.

Epidemiology Presumed to be lethal in males, although there are a few reports of affected males, several of whom had Klinefelter syndrome (47,XXY chromosome complement).

Inheritance X-linked dominant

Chromosomal location Xp11.22-p11.23

Gene EBP, coding for 3^{β}-hydroxysteroid-d^{8},d^{7}-isomerase. The gene has 5 exons in 7 kb. The transcript is 1 kb and codes for a 230 amino acid protein predicted to be an integral endoplasmic reticulum membrane protein. The human EBP gene is the homologue of the mouse gene causing the *Tattered* murine phenotype.

Mutation spectrum Missense, nonsense, splice site and frame shift mutations have been identified in a small series of 7 patients.

Effect of mutation A defect in cholesterol biosynthesis resulting in cholesterol deficiency or accumulation of a teratogenic sterol precursor is hypothesized to lead to the developmental defects in Conradi-Hunermann syndrome.

Diagnosis

Direct sequence analysis of the EBP gene from genomic DNA

Counselling issues

X-inactivation (lyonization), the turning-off of one X-chromosome in females, is a random event and is important in determining the severity of Conradi-Hunermann and other X-linked dominant disorders in affected females.

Chondrodysplasia punctata refers to the stippled epiphyses in this syndrome. This finding can occur in other disorders and there is an X-linked recessive form that also includes ichthyotic changes.

Sjögren-Larsson Syndrome

MIM

270200

Clinical features

Congenital ichthyosis with a generalized and variable distribution and quality. The skin is often very pruritic. Spastic diplegia or tetraplegia. Mental retardation. Glistening white dots on retina (in about one-third of the cases) and pigmentary retinal degeneration. Short stature. Speech delay. Seizures.

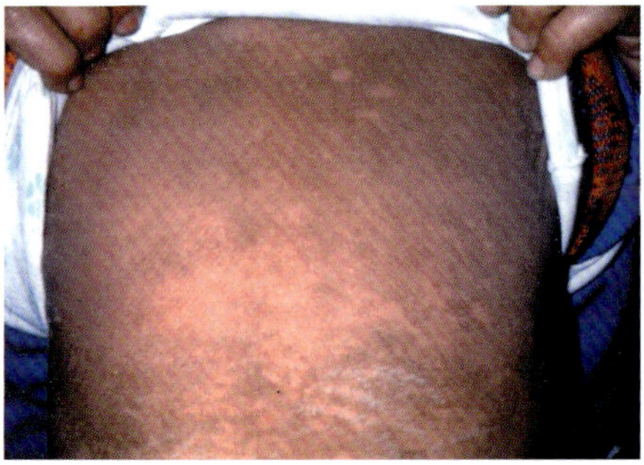

Ichthyosis in Sjögren-Larsson syndrome.

Age of onset

The ichthyosis is usually congenital, but a collodion membrane is uncommon. The neurological symptoms appear during the first or second year of life.

Epidemiology

The disorder is frequent in Sweden, where about 2% of the population is estimated to be heterozygous for the disease mutation. It has also been described in many other ethnic and racial groups.

Inheritance

Autosomal recessive

Chromosomal location

17p11.2

Gene

FALDH (also called ALDH10), coding for the enzyme fatty aldehyde dehydrogenase. The gene has 11 exons spanning 30.5 kb of genomic DNA.

Mutational spectrum

The most common Swedish mutation (also seen in other kindreds with Northern European ancestry from the Netherlands, Germany and Belgium) is a point mutation resulting in $Pro^{315}Ser$. Another relatively common mutation in Europeans is $^{1296}delGA$. Most other mutations are novel missense mutations with deletions, insertions, nonsense, splice-site and more complex rearrangements also seen. Mutations occur throughout the coding region of the gene, but there may be a clustering around nucleotide 798.

Diagnosis

Enzymatic assay of cultured amniocytes or chorionic villi cells (for prenatal diagnosis) or fibroblasts. Sequence analysis of genomic DNA or cDNA for mutations will confirm the diagnosis and allow carrier detection in family members and rapid prenatal diagnosis in subsequent at-risk pregnancies. RFLP and allele-specific PCR assays have been developed for the Swedish mutation and other more common European mutations.

Counselling issues

There is conflicting anecdotal evidence that dietary supplementation with medium-chain fatty acids may improve the cutaneous features of the disease.

Albright Hereditary Osteodystrophy

AKA

Pseudohypoparathyroidism IA

MIM

103580

Clinical features

Subcutaneous ossification developing in areas of trauma, including site of injection and pressure points such as the heel of the foot. Endocrine abnormalities including thyrotropin and gonadotropin resistance. Hypothyroidism. Mental retardation. Short stature. Short fourth and fifth metacarpals.

Age of onset

Infancy

Inheritance

Autosomal dominant, but imprinting of the GNAS1 gene (differential gene expression depending on whether the mutated gene was inherited from the mother or from the father) may play a part and contribute to the observed increased frequency of maternal inheritance.

Chromosomal location

20q13.2

Gene

GNAS1, coding for guanine nucleotide-binding protein (Gs, stimulatory). The protein is a heterotrimer.

Mutational spectrum

Mostly missense mutations, and some deletion and splice site mutations

Effect of mutation

Several mutations have been shown to lead to defective GDP-binding (increased GDP-release), thermolability and impaired receptor-mediated (decreased) activation of the GNAS1 protein. It is also suggested that tissue-specific imprinting on the GNAS1 gene is the mechanism for the variable and tissue-specific hormone resistance seen in the disorder, with the skeletal changes the result of end-organ resistance to parathyroid hormone.

Diagnosis

Both SSCP and genomic DNA sequence analysis are used to identify mutations

Counselling issues

The terminology is confusing. In pseudo-pseudohypoparathyroidism, individuals have the findings of Albright hereditary osteodystrophy, but not the hormone resistance. Pseudohypoparathyroidism IB is thought to be a receptor defect, with normal G unit activity, and only 15% of the cases having the findings of Albright hereditary osteodystrophy. Most cases of pseudohypoparathyroidism IB are sporadic. In contrast, Pseudohypoparathyroidism IA has only 50% normal G unit activity (consistent with dominant inheritance), and all cases have the findings of Albright hereditary osteodystrophy.

8. Glossary

Abbreviations

A	Adenine
ARMS	Amplification Refractory Mutation System
ASO	Allele-Specific Oligonucleotide
bp	Base Pair(s)
C	Cytosine
CDCA	Chenodeoxycholic Acid
cDNA	Complementary DNA
CF	Cystic Fibrosis
chr.	Chromosome
CHRPE	Congenital Hypertrophy of Retinal Pigment Epithelium
cM	CentiMorgan
CS	Cockayne Syndrome
CSGE	Conformation-Sensitive Gel Electrophoresis
CVS	Chorionic Villus Sampling
ddF	Di-deoxyfingerprinting
DEBD	Dominant Epidermolysis Bullosa Dystrophica
DGGE	Denaturing Gradient Gel Electrophoresis
DNA	Deoxyribonucleic Acid
ds	Double Stranded
EB	Epidermolysis Bullosa
EBS	Epidermolysis Bullosa Simplex
ECG	Electrocardiogram
EEC	Ectodermal Dysplasia-Ectrodactyly-Cleft Lip/Palate Syndrome
EHK	Epidermolytic Hyperkeratosis
EKV	Erythrokeratoderma Variabilis
EST	Expressed Sequence Tag
FAP	Familial Adenomatous Polyposis
G	Guanine
GABEB	Generalized Atrophic Benign Epidermolysis Bullosa
HANE	Hereditary Angioneurotic (O)Edema

HEP	Hepatoerythropoietic Porphyria
HHT	Hereditary Haemorrhagic Telangiectasia
HPLC	High Performance Liquid Chromatography
IBS	Ichthyosis Bullosa of Siemens
IP1	Incontinentia Pigmenti Achromians
IP2	Incontinentia Pigmenti
JEB-PA	Junctional Epidermolysis Bullosa with Pyloric Atresia
kb	Kilobase (10^3 bp of DNA)
Mb	Megabase (10^6 bp of DNA)
MHC	Major Histocompatibility Complex
MRI	Magnetic Resonance Imaging
mRNA	Messenger RNA
OCA1	Oculotaneous Albinism Type I
OCA2	Oculotaneous Albinism Type II
PC	Pachyonychia Congenita
PCR	Polymerase Chain Reaction
PCT	Porphyria Cutanea Tarda
PSEK	Progressive Symmetric Erythrokeratoderma
PTT	Protein Truncation Test
REBD	Recessive Epidermolysis Bullosa Dystrophica
RFLP	Restriction Fragment Length Polymorphism
RNA	Ribonucleic acid
RT-PCR	Reverse Transcriptase-Polymerase Chain Reaction
SER	Sarco/Endoplasmic Reticulum
ss	Single Stranded
SSCP	Single Strand Conformation Polymorphisms
STS	Sequence Tagged Site
T	Thymine
TDO	Tricho-Dento-Osseous
tRNA	Transfer RNA
TRPS	Tricho-Rhino-Phalangeal Syndrome
VNTR	Variable Number Tandem Repeats
WS	Waardenburg Syndrome
XP	Xeroderma Pigmentosum

A Matter of Scale

Human genetic disease ultimately results from changes in the sequence content of DNA. DNA is essentially a simple molecule, composed of the four bases adenine (A), thymine (T), guanine (G) and cytosine (C). It exists as a pair of anti parallel strands and has a double helical structure, as first elucidated by Watson and Crick in 1953. Adenine always pairs with thymine and guanine with cytosine, on opposite strands. The two strands of DNA are not covalently linked but attached via the hydrogen bonding that occurs between the complementary bases. Double stranded DNA (dsDNA) may be easily split into single strands by the application of heat (see Properties of DNA).

While a simple molecule, the complexity of DNA results directly from the possible sequence of its bases. Thus, a two base pair (bp) DNA molecule may have any one of $4^2 = 16$ possible sequences (the first base may be any one of the four, and, for each given first base, the second may then be any one of four). A 10 bp molecule has $4^{10} = 1{,}048{,}576$ possible sequences.

The complexity of the genome of an organism is related to its size, although there is often not a direct correlation between the complexity of a genome and that of its organism. Some plants, for example, possess genomes that are larger than that of man. In man, the size of the genome is believed to be 3×10^9 bp. This number refers to the total length of DNA in a human *haploid* genome, i.e. half the genome that is present in somatic cells. Since, apart from the sex chromosomes, all genetic material is present in two copies, the haploid figure is the more relevant, as duplication of genetic material does not increase complexity. The possible number of sequences that a length of 3×10^9 bp can generate is astronomical (4 ^ $[3 \times 10^9]$). As an example of genome complexities of different organisms, SV40, a mammalian virus, possesses 4×10^3 bp; *Escherichia coli* (*E. coli*, a bacterium) 4×10^6 bp; and *Drosophila melanogaster* (the fruit fly) 1×10^8 bp.

The complexity of the human genome is divided among 46 physically distinct chromosomes. In both sexes, there are 22 pairs of autosomes (non-sex chromosomes) plus two sex chromosomes. In the female, these are two X chromosomes, while in the male there is an X and a Y chromosome. Maleness is essentially due to the presence of the Y chromosome. An average human chromosome contains about 100 megabases (Mb) of DNA, although this number varies as human chromosomes vary widely in size. Human chromosome 21 , for example, is one of the smallest and has a length of 50 Mb, while chromosome 1 has 300 Mb (chromosomes are numbered inversely according to their size, 1 being the largest).

Recently, the full sequence of the euchromatic (i.e. coding) portion of human chromosome 22 has been published — the published length is approximately 33 Mb. This represents the first in a series of landmarks associated with the international effort to sequence the entire human genome — the Human Genome Project.

Figure 1 is a standard representation of a normal (male) human karyotype, illustrating the size range of human chromosomes.

Figure 1. Schematic of a normal human (male) karyotype. (ISCN 550 ideogram produced by the MRC Human Genetics Unit, Edinburgh, reproduced with permission)

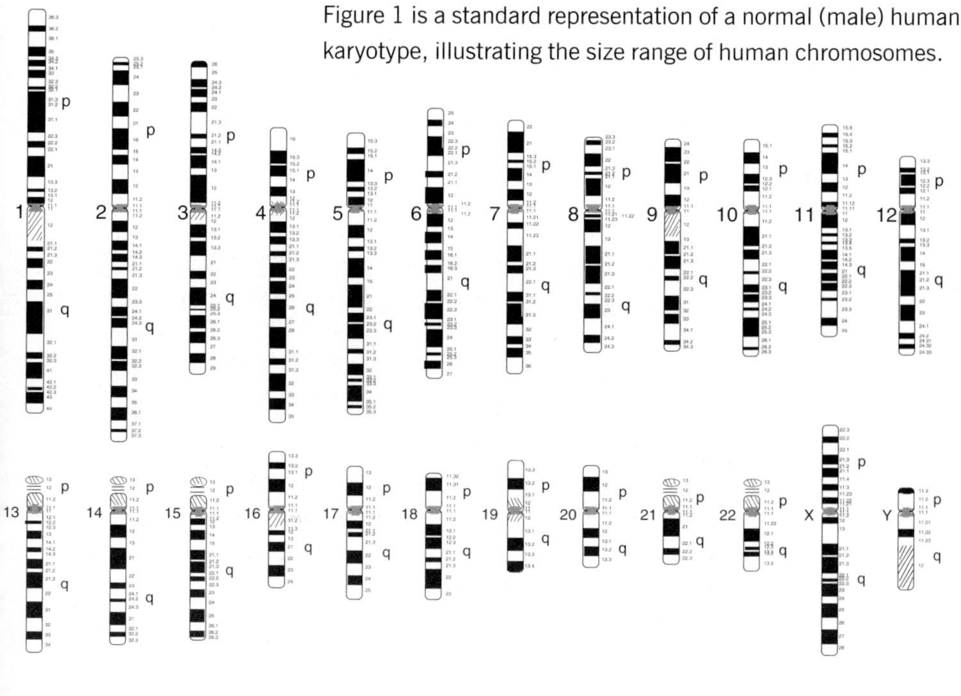

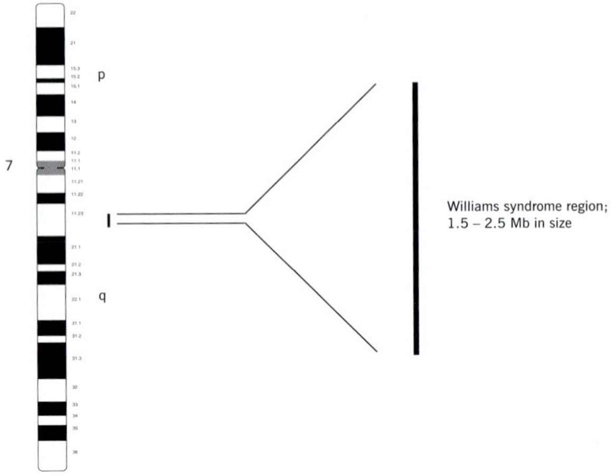

Figure 2. Schematic demonstrating the common deletion found in Williams syndrome at 7q11.23 (see text).

Figure 2 gives some idea of the size of an individual chromosome, in this example chromosome 7. Williams syndrome is a sporadic disorder associated with a heterozygous deletion of between 1.5-2.5 Mb of DNA. Despite the absence of such a long stretch of DNA (thought to contain over 15 genes), the deletion cannot be routinely detected by cytogenetic examination alone, due to its relatively small size (i.e. by cytogenetic standards). Demonstration of this deletion relies on the use of FISH analysis.

Mutations and genetic disease

A vast range of different mutations have been described in association with human genetic disease. In general, it is not possible to correlate the severity of a mutation with that of the concomitant disease. Single base substitutions may cause very severe phenotypes, while certain individuals who harbour gross cytogenetic rearrangements (e.g. resulting in genomic imbalance) may be phenotypically normal.

Until recently, mutations were believed to represent all-or-none phenomena. A number of different conditions are now known to be associated with dynamic mutations and, in this category of condition, there is, broadly speaking, a correlation between mutation severity and disease severity.

The following is a brief description of the types of mutation that are found in association with human genetic disease.

Non-dynamic mutations

This category (the majority) encompasses all the possible mutations that are essentially stable; if transmitted, the offspring will possess the same mutation. In many cases, however, a mutation may be genetically lethal, i.e. it causes reproductive failure in the most general sense of the word. In some conditions, the failure to reproduce results exclusively from physical abnormalities (e.g. azoospermia in Klinefelter's syndrome), while in others the reasons are primarily social (e.g. Rett syndrome, a severe mental retardation syndrome affecting girls almost exclusively). Females with classical Rett syndrome do not reproduce for obvious social reasons but probably have normal fertility.

A. Single base substitutions

Single base substitutions, also known as point mutations, are the best characterised of all mutations. The Cardiff Human Gene Mutation Database (http://www.uwcm.ac.uk/uwcm/mg/hgmd0.html) is a repository of human gene mutations and keeps an up to date record of all reported mutations, in a variety of categories. The vast majority of point mutations are missense or nonsense mutations. These alter a codon so that either a different amino acid is encoded (missense) or a codon used to specify an amino acid in a normal individual now specifies a stop codon (nonsense), resulting in premature termination of the protein.

Point mutations may also affect splicing, the process by which mature messenger RNA (mRNA) is produced from RNA that has been transcribed directly off the chromosome, or the regulation of genes (either positively or negatively).

B. Small deletions/insertions

Almost 5000 entries in the Cardiff Human Gene Mutation Database attest to this relatively common mode of mutation, in which up to 20 bp of DNA are either deleted or inserted. Such insertions/deletions almost always alter the reading frame of the gene, resulting in a frame shift mutation and premature termination of the reading frame of the gene.

A well known example of this mutational type is the frequent mutation found in patients with cystic fibrosis. The mutation, known as ΔF508 (deletion of codon 508, encoding F - phenylalanine), is actually an exception to the general rule that insertions/deletions generally alter the reading frame. Because exactly 3 bases are deleted, the rest of the gene is in frame.

C. Submicroscopic genomic rearrangements (microdeletions/microduplications)

Until recently, the importance of this category of mutation in human genetic disease was grossly underestimated. It is now appreciated that many patients, particularly those with complex physical/intellectual abnormalities, have cytogenetically undetectable deletions/insertions/translocations that nevertheless have serious phenotypic consequences. Since the limit of cytogenetic resolution, even in the best laboratories, is of the order of 5 Mb of DNA, in many patients with rearrangements involving a smaller amount of material than this the causative lesion is likely to be missed. A good example is Williams syndrome. This sporadic disorder was first described in the 1960s and presents with a mixture of physical and developmental abnormalities. Patients (males and females are equally affected) have moderate learning difficulties and specific cardiac (supravalvular aortic stenosis - SVAS) and biochemical (hypercalcaemia in infancy) abnormalities. Despite intensive investigation by many laboratories, no reports of consistent cytogenetic abnormalities were ever reported.
The only clue to the aetiology of this condition came from the analysis of a family segregating a balanced translocation between chromosomes 6 and 7, in whom SVAS was present in every carrier of the rearrangement. It was subsequently demonstrated that the translocation interrupted the elastin gene on chromosome 7

(at 7q11.23 - see Figure 2). Use of the elastin gene as a DNA probe for FISH analysis revealed that approximately 98% of individuals with this condition had only one copy of the gene. It could be argued that without the serendipitous discovery of the translocation family, the cause of Williams syndrome would still be unknown. The diagnosis of Williams syndrome is now a routine matter and performed in many laboratories.

Williams syndrome is an example of a haplo-insufficiency disorder; one that results from reduced, rather than absent, gene expression. Many other conditions are now known to result from the same general mechanism, and it is suspected that a large proportion of patients who present with complex physical/intellectual abnormalities but who have normal karyotypes may have haplo-insufficiency of large regions of their genomes.

In recent years it has become clear that the mechanism whereby a large segment of the genome is deleted depends on the presence of chromosome-specific repeat units (see Figure 3). This mechanism also results in the creation of a complementary mutation, namely the duplication, and there are at least two examples

Figure 3. Schematic demonstrating (i) normal homologous recombination and (ii) homologous unequal recombination, resulting in a deletion and a duplication chromosome.

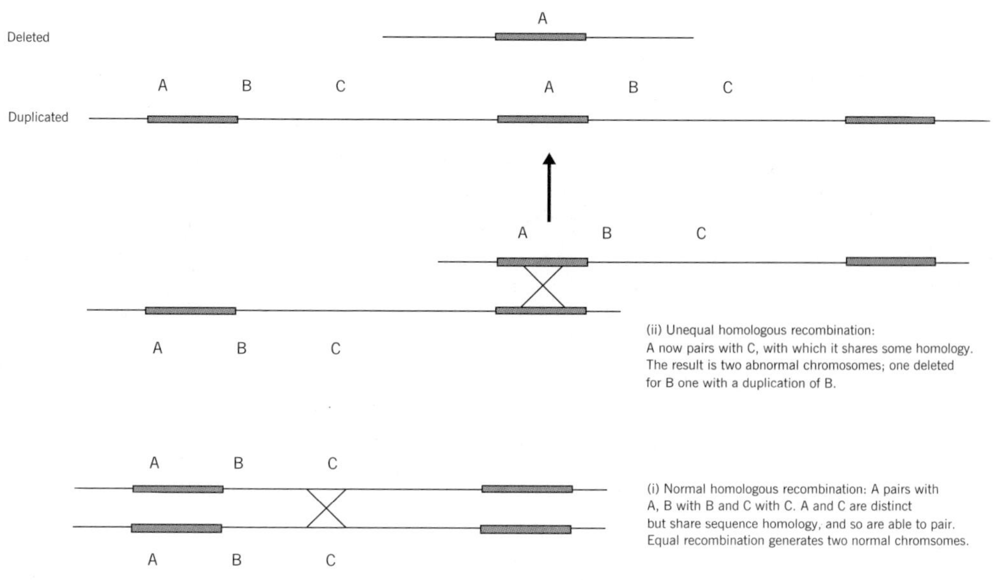

where both the deletion and its reciprocal duplication have been described as causing distinct phenotypes (one example is Charcot-Marie-Tooth type 1A [duplication at 17p11.2] and its counterpart hereditary neuropathy with liability to pressure palsies - HNPP [deletion at 17p11.2]).

D. Cytogenetically visible rearrangements

Individuals with cytogenetically visible rearrangements (deletions/inversions/duplications/translocations) generally have severe phenotypes, if there is imbalance, although exceptions do exist. Genomic imbalance is generally not well tolerated and only a small fraction of all possible imbalances are ever observed, presumably because the others are lethal to the individual.

For example, only three trisomies are commonly observed, namely those involving chromosomes 21 (Down syndrome), 18 (Edwards syndrome) and 13 (Patau syndrome). Other trisomies are observed but very rarely and often only in a mosaic state (i.e. the individual possesses normal cells in addition to cells that carry an additional chromosome). Interestingly, monosomy (i.e. compete absence of one of a pair of homologous chromosomes) is extremely rare, except in Turner syndrome, 45XO.

Deletions or duplications of chromosomal segments are frequently observed in individuals with learning difficulties and physical abnormalities.

In all cases of genomic imbalance, it is very difficult to correlate precisely the size of the imbalance and the phenotype, although in general a smaller imbalance is better than a larger one. With the exception of patients with microdeletions, for which a common mutational mechanism often results in the same deletion in many different individuals, the gross deletions that are observed cytogenetically are likely to all be unique. In other words, a seemingly identical deletion of a chromosomal segment in two patients is likely to differ markedly at the molecular level. For this reason it is difficult to counsel accurately in such situations.

It is not entirely clear why genomic imbalance is so detrimental. Classical thinking in genetics has always focused on the phenotypic consequences of absent gene expression, but the description in recent years of a range of disorders associated with haplo-insufficiency (in particular) or increased expression has forced a dramatic alteration of this view, particularly in human genetics. One possible explanation is that because of the complexity of human beings and our (relatively) sophisticated ability to define phenotypic variation, many more phenotypes are possible in man, than even our closest primate relatives. After all, would a monkey with Williams syndrome (who survived the cardiac abnormality) be noticed? Moderate learning difficulties and a special talent for music hardly seem relevant! Because of the range of phenotypes that we can clinically name, any subtle alteration in the genetic program is likely to be noticed. Another way of thinking about the imbalance issue is that a 240V television would probably not work at 120V, and at 360V, might explode or produce a picture and sound that was highly distorted. Our evolution has always occurred on the template of diploidy and has taken that for granted, so that imbalance in either direction is likely to be deleterious.

Properties of DNA

Despite the existence of a plethora of techniques designed to analyse DNA, the essential properties of DNA upon which such techniques are based are relatively few.

DNA normally exists as a double-stranded (ds) molecule, containing two strands that are complementary in sequence. The two strands are joined by hydrogen bonding, a non-covalent mechanism that is easily reversible using heat or chemical means. Thus, if one strand of DNA is known to possess the sequence 5′-CCGGATCGT-3′ (5′ and 3′ refer to the numbering of carbons on the deoxyribose ring; the convention is to write down the sequence of DNA in a 5′→3′ direction), then the sequence of its complement can be immediately deduced, as C always pairs with G and A with T:

5′ - CCGGATCGT - 3′

3′ - GGCCTAGCA - 5′

Note that the complementary sequence is written 3′→5′, as it is upside-down.

In dsDNA, each strand contains the same information as the full molecule, and can serve as a template for synthesis of the dsDNA structure. This is the basis of DNA replication, the mechanism by which DNA is copied.

Finally, and most importantly, single strands of DNA that possess complementary sequences can find each other in a complex mixture of molecules and re-anneal with high specificity. This phenomenon of re-annealing or re-association, is based on the stability of perfectly matched sequences and the instability of imperfectly matched ones. dsDNA that is melted into single-stranded form by, for example, heating will re-associate at a rate that depends on the sequence complexity of the starting material. Thus, a given mass of DNA originating from a simple genome (say a virus) will re-anneal much faster than the same mass originating from the human genome. The greater the complexity of the starting material, the lower the concentration of each unique entity within the mix. Much research has been conducted on the precise mechanism of DNA re-association, as well as the kinetics involved. For the purpose of a basic understanding of many of the techniques of molecular biology that rely on this phenomenon, it suffices to think of the mechanism as follows.

In a complex mix of single-stranded DNA molecules, molecules bump into each other continuously. When short stretches of complementarity find each other in solution, the structure that results will possess a certain stability dependent on the length of complementarity. In practice, most such experiments are conducted at relatively high temperatures (e.g. 65°C), so that only true matches are stable (the higher the temperature, the less stable are short regions of complementarity). When two single-stranded molecules interact at a short region of complementarity, the interaction is likely to be brief unless flanking sequences are also complementary. When two molecules that have significant lengths of sequence complementarity interact, a zippering mechanism is believed to follow the initial seed or short stretch of complementarity. The zippering mechanism rapidly ensures greater stability of the newly formed dsDNA molecule, which will remain in ds form unless heat/chemical treatment is re-applied.

This sequence-specific re-association is the basis for most of the currently used techniques of molecular biology. In Southern blotting, for example, the DNA that is being interrogated is immobilised in single-stranded form on a solid support, such as a nitrocellulose membrane. The DNA used as a probe is also single-stranded, and is radioactively labelled. The two are mixed and allowed to re-anneal. The probe will interact with all the molecules on the membrane but will only remain stably bound to those that are complementary in sequence — the specificity of Southern blotting is directly related to the specificity of DNA re-association. In PCR, short oligonucleotides are used to prime DNA synthesis from specific sites in the genome — annealing of these oligonucleotides occurs in much the same way. The first step in PCR always involves melting the DNA to be amplified and allowing the oligonucleotides (which are single-stranded) to anneal to the DNA (see Commonly Used Techniques for more information).

Commonly Used Techniques

1. Southern and Northern blotting
2. Polymerase chain reaction (PCR)
3. PCR based methods:
    a. Deletion screening
    b. Use of mRNA/cDNA
    c. Single-strand conformation polymorphism analysis (SSCP)
    d. Sequencing
    e. Rapid screening for known mutations
4. DNA chips
5. Cytogenetics and in situ hybridisation (ISH/FISH)

Southern and Northern blotting

The technique of Southern blotting, so named for its inventor (Southern, 1975), paved the way for direct analysis of specific genes in a complex mixture. Genomic DNA is cleaved with a restriction enzyme (an endonuclease that will only digest DNA at specific sequences). The size range of DNA fragments generated depends on the site recognised by the enzyme. For example, enzymes that recognise 4 bp sites cleave, on average, more frequently than those that recognise 6 bp sites, and therefore generate a larger number of fragments, with a shorter average length. The digested DNA may be size fractionated on an agarose gel and then transferred to a membrane, which acts as a solid support. The membrane, with its bound DNA, can subsequently be used in experiments with specific DNA sequences as probes.

The basic approach to Southern blotting is illustrated in Figure 4.

Northern blotting refers to essentially the same process, except that RNA is the transferred nucleic acid. Northern blotting is so named in order to differentiate it from Southern blotting, and not because

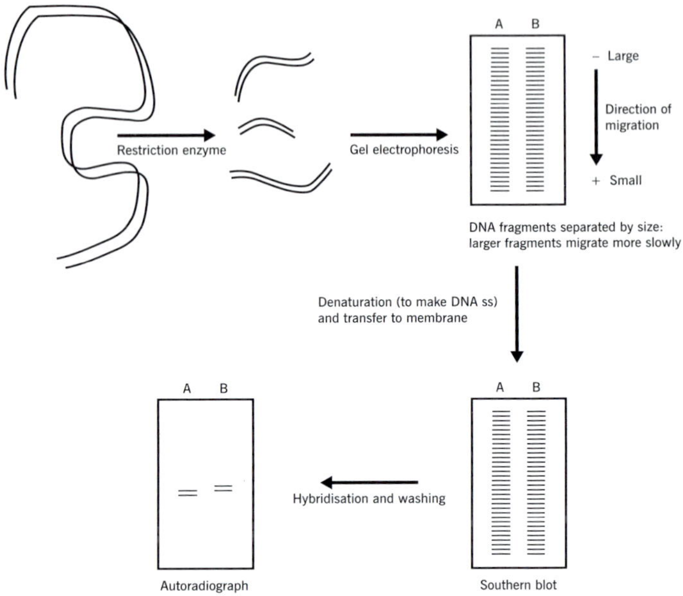

Figure 4. Southern blotting. High molecular weight genomic DNA is digested, using a restriction enzyme, which cleaves at specific sites. The cleaved fragments are resolved by gel electrophoresis, on the basis of size. The sizes of fragments generated are essentially random, although the range of sizes is dependent on the frequency of appearance of the recognised site in the genome (the longer the recognition sequence, the less often it appears in the genome and the larger the average fragment size). After gel electrophoresis, the DNA is denatured to make it single stranded (i.e., with alkali treatment) and transferred to a 'solid' support, such as a nitrocellulose membrane. This Southern blot can then be used in hybridisation experiments with radiolabelled DNA sequences of interest, which specifically bind to regions of the blot that contain complementary sequences.

any specific direction is implied.

While standard Southern blotting has been used for DNA fractionated using conventional gels, it has also been applied to the fractionation of gels using pulsed field gel electrophoresis, a technique that allows for the fractionation of very large DNA molecules

Polymerase chain reaction (PCR)

PCR was first described by Saiki et al. in 1985. The technique involves the *in vitro* amplification of specific DNA sequences. PCR has revolutionised the way in which both research genetics and diagnostic work is carried out and has almost totally obviated the need for Southern blotting (although blots are still required for specific situations such as genomic rearrangements).

The principle of PCR is simple: genomic DNA is repeatedly copied, using short stretches of DNA that have been synthesised specifically for the purpose (primers or oligonucleotides) and a

DNA polymerase. The primers bind to genomic DNA at a site complementary to their sequence and the polymerase then synthesises DNA complementary to the sequence adjacent to the primer.

Standard PCR involves repeated cycles of *three* main steps (see Figure 5.)

1. Heat denaturation — this makes the DNA to be copied single-stranded and usually occurs at 95°C

2. Annealing of primers — the temperature at which this takes place will depend on the specific primer sequences but generally occurs in the range of 50-65°C

3. Extension of the annealed primers with DNA polymerase — thermostable DNA polymerases are used, which can withstand repeated rounds of high temperatures without significant loss of activity. These enzymes are isolated from thermophilic bacteria, which have evolved to survive at high temperatures

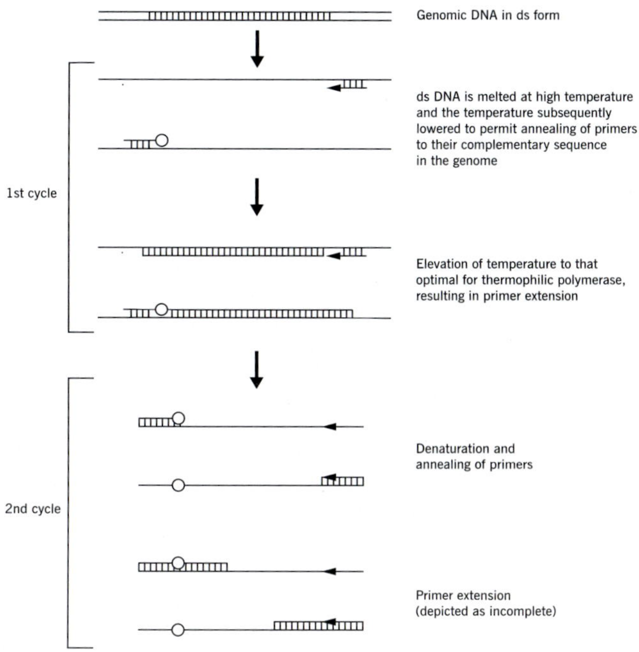

Figure 5. Schematic illustrating the technique of polymerase chain reaction (PCR). Genomic DNA is melted into ss form, primers are annealed to specific regions in the genome, and primer extension is performed with a thermophilic polymerase. After the first cycle, the primers anneal to both the original genomic DNA template, as well as newly synthesised DNA strands. PCR results in exponential amplification of DNA, the theoretical yield being 2^n times the starting material, where n is the number of cycles performed.

in their environment

The effect of PCR is that each round results in a doubling of the DNA sequences present in the previous round. This results in an exponential increase in the copy number of the specific sequences being amplified. Traditionally, a PCR reaction takes a few hours to complete but recent improvements in technology mean that, with some thermal cyclers, the reaction can be completed in 20-30 minutes.

Additional improvements in PCR have meant that longer products can be generated (up to 40 kb, whereas standard PCR typically only generates products of less than 1 kb). PCR has made realistic the goal of same-day diagnosis and is now an indispensable tool in diagnostic labs. PCR also forms the basis of many techniques for mutation detection.

PCR-based methods of mutation detection

The advent of PCR has made the detection of many mutations in human genetic disease both straightforward and rapid. While PCR is used universally, there exist situations where the older method of Southern blotting is still desirable (e.g. detection of gross genomic rearrangements).

In some cases, the gene of interest is so large, and the range of mutations so wide, that a variety of approaches are required when mutations in that gene are suspected (e.g. the dystrophin gene in Duchenne muscular dystrophy).

The following is a list of commonly used techniques that are based on PCR. It is not exhaustive but contains most of the important approaches currently in use.

Deletion screening

This approach is most suitable for situations in which a DNA sequence is totally absent from the patient being investigated. Thus, in Duchenne muscular dystrophy (DMD), deletions are often found. A multiplex PCR can be carried out, in which amplification

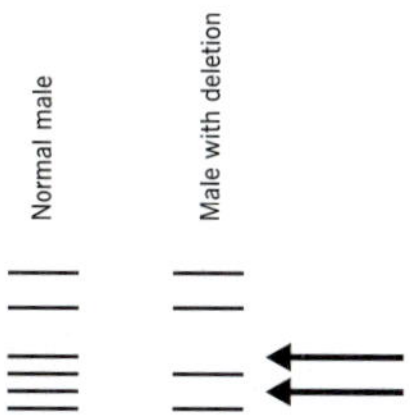

Figure 6. Schematic of multiplex DNA amplification of 6 fragments from the Duchenne muscular dystrophy gene. All six bands are present in the normal male control; the affected patient had two bands missing (arrowed), consistent with deletion.

of a number of exons of the dystrophin gene is performed simultaneously. Since males have only one copy of the dystrophin gene, any deletion of sequences from this gene will result in failure to amplify that sequence (i.e. the result is all or none). This is demonstrated in Figure 6. The presence of fragments amplified from non-deleted regions of the gene serves as a positive control for the sequence that has failed to amplify.

Deletion analysis can be carried out for heterozygous carriers of deletion mutations but the results are not as straightforward, and dosage analysis is required in order to determine whether the PCR product is reduced by 50%.

Use of mRNA/cDNA as diagnostic material

In theory, the use of cDNA (DNA that has been generated from mRNA and is complementary in sequence to it) is a preferred method for the detection of mutations. In addition to being more direct, the length of nucleic acid that must be analysed is much less than is the case for the relevant genomic equivalent of the gene (e.g. the dystrophin gene spans 2.4 Mb of genomic DNA but its transcript is only about 14 kb long). Direct examination of cDNA also allows detection of splicing mutations, namely those that affect the way transcribed RNA is converted to mature mRNA. The major drawback of cDNA analysis is that the gene of interest may not be expressed in tissues that are easily accessible (such as blood). While biopsy of the relevant organ is possible (e.g. muscle in the case of DMD), this approach is not always desirable. In some cases, however, it may be possible to amplify very low levels of ectopic transcripts and analyse these (this has been done in a number of situations; e.g. factor VIII transcripts have been amplified from peripheral white cells, whereas the major site of transcription is the liver).

Single-strand conformation polymorphism analysis (SSCP)

The electrophoretic mobility of a single-stranded DNA molecule is a function not only of its size but also its nucleotide sequence.

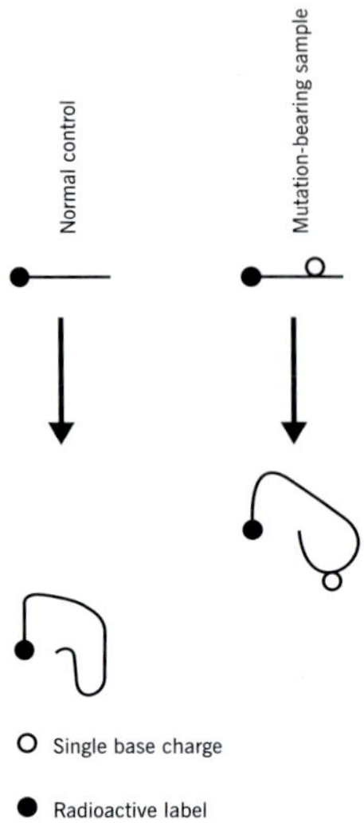

Figure 7. PCR products are generated from normal controls and patient samples; one strand is end-labelled, the dsDNA product is melted and the DNA run on a non-denaturing gel, so as to allow the single strands to adopt a secondary stucture. The presence of a single base alteration is sufficient, in the majority of cases, to alter the secondary structure, and hence the mobility of the fragment, so that a difference is discernable in band pattern between controls and patients.

Under non-denaturing conditions, single-stranded DNA molecules do not exist as linear molecules but rather fold up into conformations that depend on size, sequence and ionic conditions. Thus a single base substitution may alter the mobility of a single-stranded DNA molecule, even though there is relatively little alteration in mass. In a variety of studies, over 90% of mutations were detectable using SSCP. The advantage of the method is its simplicity, although in some cases some optimisation of running conditions is required to detect certain mutations.

Briefly, one strand of the DNA to be studied (invariably a PCR product) is radioactively labelled, and then the sample is run on a non-denaturing gel (i.e. the single strands are allowed to fold up). Single-base substitutions are detectable by shifts in mobility of the samples with respect to normal controls (see Figure 7).

SSCP is an effective screening tool for initial detection of mutations, although because it is not 100% effective, other approaches must be combined when exhaustive searches are required.

Sequencing

Direct DNA sequencing may be used both in initial searches for causative mutations and for confirmation of mutations detected using other methods, such as SSCP. PCR products may be sequenced directly, or first cloned into a vector. The latter approach is more time consuming and may generate artefacts related to PCR or the cloning step. Direct sequencing of PCR products in heterozygous individuals will typically produce an ambiguity at the site of mutation — the wild-type base will coincide with the mutated base at that position.

Rapid screening when the mutation is known

In many cases, great effort is expended in initial detection of the causative mutation in an individual patient. Once the mutation is known, however, subsequent analysis in relatives of that patient is much more straightforward. In addition to direct sequencing, other methods may be employed. Allele-specific oligonucleotides (ASOs) may be used in PCR; oligonucleotides are designed that incorporate the mutated base. Under the right conditions, they will only prime amplification when their precise counterpart is present. In this way, mutated and wild-type alleles can be differentiated.

A point mutation may generate/abolish a restriction site for an available enzyme. PCR across the point mutation results in a product that will either cleave or be resistant to cleavage depending on the mutation that has occurred.

In many diseases, a single mutation is causative in the majority of patients and simple screening tests can be used whenever this disease is encountered. In some diseases, the mutation is always the same. In sickle cell disease, for example, only one mutation is involved. In others, one mutation accounts for the majority (e.g. cystic fibrosis).

In many conditions, however, the range of mutations is great and other approaches are in development that allow for simultaneous detection of the mutations.

DNA chips

It was inevitable that the digital age would have an impact on genetics. Much work has been done in the last few years to develop DNA chips, both as research tools and for diagnostic use. While DNA chips, strictly speaking, refer to silicon-based chips on which short stretches of DNA (oligonucleotides) are generated using a photolithographic process, the term has also been used generally to refer to any small array of DNA sequences, whether produced as just described or resulting from spotting of much longer DNA sequences onto glass slides.

In the diagnostic field, DNA chips have been produced to address the mutation detection problem in a number of diseases. An example is the BRCA1 chip, which was designed specifically for mutation detection in that gene. Briefly, the chip was created by a photolithographic process and contained over 96,000 oligonucleotide sequences. The oligonucleotides were designed to reflect both the wild-type sequence and also a range of possible mutations, including all possible single base substitutions and a variety of small deletions or insertions. Analysis is carried out by labelling patient samples with one fluorescent tag (e.g. red) and a wild-type control with another tag (e.g. green). Sequences in the patient and wild-type samples that hybridise equally to a given oligonucleotide give equal intensities in the red and green channels, while those sequences present only in one of the samples will generate an increased signal in that channel (e.g. a mutation present in the patient will generate a predominantly red signal on the complementary oligonucleotide). The power of the chip/array approach results from massive parallel processing. In practice, chips designed to detect mutations in specific genes work well, in one case detecting 14/15 known mutations. The drawbacks include the huge number of oligonucleotides required to detect all possible mutations that might occur. In some cases, many more than one chip is required to scan all exons of a gene. It is likely, however, that the technology will improve and greater oligonucleotide densities will become possible.

Cytogenetics and in situ hybridisation

It was not until 1956 that it was demonstrated that humans possess 46 chromosomes; until that time the number had been thought to be 48. Within a short time after that demonstration by Tijo and Levan, the chromosomal basis of a number of conditions was recognised, including Down syndrome (trisomy 21), Turner syndrome (45XO) and Klinefelter syndrome (47, XXY).

Improvements in cytogenetics have resulted in the process becoming both routine and more powerful, although, as explained below, there are still important limitations to the power of routine cytogenetics.

The analysis of chromosome number and morphology is still the mainstay in a range of clinical situations and the challenge for non-specialists is in deciding when a karyotype should be requested. Most abnormalities that can be detected by even the highest resolution cytogenetics will involve at least 5 Mb of genetic material. As a rule of thumb, therefore, cytogenetic investigation is not warranted when the genetic lesion is suspected to be significantly smaller than this threshold. In practice, however, a karyotype is often a good screening procedure, particularly where no clear clinical diagnosis is available to point to a specific test.

In recent years, the techniques of in situ hybridisation (ISH) and, in particular fluorescent in situ hybridisation (FISH) have allowed for a narrowing of the gulf that lies between cytogenetics and molecular genetics. While cytogenetics typically works at the 5 Mb (5×10^6) level, and molecular genetics typically at the 1 kb (10^3) level, FISH allows lesions to be detected that lie between these two ranges. Thus, it is now known that many conditions result from deletions of 1-2 Mb of material — a size of deletion considered sub-microscopic (i.e. below the level of resolution of high resolution cytogenetics). Such deletions can be clearly demonstrated using FISH. Briefly, a DNA sequence (usually a cosmid of approximately 40 kb) is labelled using a fluorescent tag and hybridized to a glass slide containing chromosomes from the patient under investigation. In the case of a deletion spanning 1-2 Mb, and a cosmid derived from the deleted sequence, a signal will only be detected on one chromosome, clearly illustrating the presence of the deletion on one chromosome and not the other. The major difference between FISH and cytogenetics is that no prior suspicion of the location of the lesion is required in cytogenetics — in other words cytogenetics is a screening procedure that will detect large enough rearrangements wherever they occur. In FISH, however, a strong clinical suspicion of a particular syndrome is required before the test can be performed, as a specific DNA sequence must be used for the test.

Cytogenetics and the artistry associated with it are likely to still have a role in the future for certain applications, however, the advent of DNA chips/microarrays may soon herald the end of the era of cytogenetics, in much the same way that PCR has largely overtaken Southern blotting. The availability of densely packed DNA chips containing genome wide sequences, for which map information is known, will make the task of searching for genomic imbalance in patients both more straightforward and reproducible.

Explanation of Terms

Alleles	Alternative forms of a DNA sequence at a given location. May apply to coding or non-coding sequences
Amniocentesis	Withdrawal of amniotic fluid for the purpose of prenatal diagnosis. This is usually carried out during the second trimester
Amplification	Production of increased numbers of copies of a DNA sequence
Aneuploid	The number of chromosomes is not an exact multiple of the haploid chromosome number. For example, patients with Trisomy 21 have one extra chromosome present in each cell; i.e. they possess 47 chromosomes in each cell
Autosome	Any chromosome other than the sex chromosomes (X or Y) or the mitochondrial chromosome
Autosomal disorder	Disorder related to an autosomal gene
Barr body	Inactive X chromosome, visible in the somatic cells of individuals with more than one X chromosome (e.g. all normal females, and males with Klinefelter's syndrome). For individuals with n X chromosomes, n-1 Barr bodies are seen
Base pair (bp)	Basic unit for measuring DNA length comprising one hydrogen-bonded pair of nucleotides. Guanine always pairs with cytosine, and thymine always pairs with adenine
Carrier	An individual who is heterozygous for a mutant allele (i.e. who carries one normal and one mutated copy of the gene under consideration). In recessive disorders, the phenotype is usually only manifest in the homozygous state
centiMorgan (cM)	The unit of genetic distance. If the chance of recombination between two loci is 1%, the loci are said to be 1 cM apart. On average, 1 cM implies a physical distance of 1 Mb, but significant deviations from this rule of thumb occur because recombination frequencies vary throughout the genome. Thus, if recombination in a certain region is less likely than

average, 1 cM may be equivalent to 5 Mb in that region

Centromere Central constriction of the chromosome, separating the short (p) from the long (q) arms

Chorionic villus sampling (CVS) Prenatal diagnostic procedure for obtaining foetal tissue at an earlier stage of gestation than amniocentesis. Generally performed after 10 weeks, ultrasound is used to guide aspiration of tissue from the villus area of the chorion

Chromatids The two identical, parallel strands of the doubled chromosome, which are connected at the centromere

Chromosomal disorders Disorders that result from gross changes in chromosome dose. May result from addition or loss of entire chromosomes, or just portions of chromosomes

Clone Group of genetically identical cells with a common ancestor

Codon Triplet of 3 bases in DNA or RNA, encoding a specific amino acid

Complementary DNA (cDNA) DNA synthesized from mRNA, using reverse transcriptase. Differs from the genomic DNA that encodes the gene of interest because of lack of introns

Compound heterozygote Individual with two different mutant alleles at the same locus

Concordant Twin pair in which both individuals manifest the same phenotype

Conformation sensitive gel electrophoresis The separation of heteroduplexes (mixtures of two species of DNA) from homoduplexes (DNA with the same sequence) containing single base-pair differences using a polyacrylamide gel

Consanguinity Sharing a common ancestor, and thus genetically related

Consultand Individual seeking genetic advice

Crossing over Reciprocal exchange of genetic material between homologous chromosomes at meiosis

Cytotrophoblasts Cells obtained from foetal chorionic villi by CVS; used for DNA and chromosome analysis

Degeneracy of the genetic code	Several codons specifying the same amino acid. This is inevitable if one considers that there are $4^3 = 64$ different possible codons and only 20 amino acids
Diploid	Number of chromosomes in most somatic cells (for humans = 46). This is double the number found in gametes (the haploid number)
Discordant	Twin pair in which the individuals differ in manifestation of a phenotype
Dizygotic	The result of fertilisation of two separate eggs by two separate sperm. Genetically non-identical twin pair
DNA (deoxyribonucleic acid)	The molecule of heredity
DNA methylation	Modification of certain nucleotides of DNA with a methyl group. In humans, the modification usually involves the cytosine that resides in the sequence CG. Methylation is associated with reduced levels of expression of a given gene and is important in imprinting
Dominant	Manifesting a phenotype in the heterozygous state. Thus, individuals with Huntington's chorea, a dominant condition, are affected even though they possess one normal copy of the gene
Empirical recurrence risks	Information for relatives based on observation, rather than detailed knowledge of modes of inheritance, environmental factors, etc.
Endonuclease	An enzyme that cleaves DNA at an internal site. Restriction endonucleases (restriction enzymes) cleave DNA at specific sites, determined by the DNA sequence
Euchromatin	Chromatin that stains lightly with trypsin G banding and contains active/potentially active genes
Exons	The coding parts of a gene. Exons are found in mature mRNA, whereas introns are not
Expressivity	Degree of expression of a disease. Autosomal dominant disorders are often associated with variable expressivity
Familial	Any trait that has a higher frequency in relatives of an affected individual than in the general population

Founder effect	High frequency of a mutant allele in a population as a result of its presence in a founder (ancestor)
Frameshift mutation	Deletion/insertion of a DNA sequence that is not an exact multiple of 3 bp. The result is an alteration of the reading frame of the gene such that the entire sequence that lies beyond the mutation is effectively nonsense. It is usually the case that a stop codon is encountered shortly after the frameshift
Gamete	Mature sex cell (the ovum of the female or the spermatozoon of the male)
Genetic code	The matrix that assigns to each codon either a specific amino acid or an instruction (start/stop)
Genetic counselling	Information/advice given to families with, or at risk of, genetic disease
Genetic heterogeneity	Association of a specific phenotype with mutations at different loci. The broader the phenotypic criteria, the greater the heterogeneity (e.g. mental retardation). Even very specific phenotypes, however, may be genetically heterogeneous (e.g. tuberous sclerosis). Not to be confused with allelic heterogeneity, which refers to the presence of different mutations at the same locus. Locus heterogeneity refers to mutations at different loci
Genetically lethal	Prevents reproduction. Not necessarily lethal to the individual concerned (e.g. females with Turner's syndrome)
Genetic locus	A specific location on a chromosome
Genetic marker	A locus that can be detected. May represent anonymous DNA or a gene sequence
Genetic screening	Population analysis designed to ascertain individuals at risk of either suffering or transmitting a genetic disease
Genome	The complete DNA sequence of an individual. The genome of humans is estimated to have a complexity of 3.3×10^9 bp (per haploid genome)
Genomic	Pertaining to the genome. Genomic DNA differs from cDNA

in that it contains non-coding as well as coding DNA

Genotype Genetic constitution of an individual

Giemsa banding Light/dark bar code obtained by staining chromosomes with Giemsa stain. Results in a unique bar code for each chromosome

Haploid The chromosome number of a normal gamete, containing one each of every individual chromosome (= 23 in humans)

Haplotype Genotype of a group of alleles from two or more closely linked loci on one chromosome. Often applied to anonymous DNA markers, occasionally to genes

Heterochromatin Darkly staining with Giemsa and mostly composed of repetitive DNA

Heterozygous Presence of two different alleles at a given locus

Histones Proteins bound to DNA in chromosomes. Functionally important in DNA activity

Homozygous Presence of identical alleles at a given locus

Hybridisation (or re-annealing) Pairing of complementary strands of nucleic acid. May also be used to refer to fusion of two somatic cells, resulting in a hybrid that contains genetic information from both donors

In situ hybridisation Annealing of DNA sequences to immobilised chromosomes. Historically done using radioactively labelled DNA; currently most often performed with fluorescently tagged molecules (fluorescent in situ hybridisation - FISH)

Index case Proband

Insertion Interruption of a chromosomal sequence as a result of insertion of material from elsewhere in the genome (either a different chromosome, or elsewhere from the same chromosome)

Intron Non-coding DNA sequence between exons. Removed from transcribed RNA by a process known as splicing

Inversion Reversal of a chromosomal segment. Pericentric inversions involve the centromere; paracentric ones do not

Karyotype — An individual's chromosome constitution, listing the number of chromosomes, sex chromosome status and any abnormalities of chromosome number or morphology

Kilobase (kb) — 1000 bp of DNA

Linkage — Co-inheritance of DNA sequences as a result of physical proximity on a chromosome. Unlinked sequences are co-inherited at an average rate of 50% because of recombination at meiosis. For linked sequences, the closer they lie to each other, the less likely they are to be separated by recombination and the more likely they are to be inherited as a single unit

Linkage disequilibrium — Association of particular DNA sequences with each other more often than is likely by chance alone. Of particular relevance to inbred populations (e.g. as in Finland), where specific disease mutations are found to reside in close proximity to specific variants of DNA markers as a result of the founder effect

Linkage map — Map of genetic markers as determined by *genetic* analysis (e.g. recombination analysis). May differ markedly from a map determined by actual physical relationships of genetic markers because of the variability of recombination

Locus heterogeneity — Mutations at different loci causing the same phenotype

LOD (logarithm of the odds) score — Statistical test of linkage, used to determine whether a result is likely to have occurred by chance or to truly reflect linkage. The LOD score is the logarithm (base 10) of the likelihood that the linkage is meaningful. A LOD score of 3 implies that there exists only a 1:1000 possibility of the results occurring by chance, and is taken as proof of linkage (i.e. the result would be likely to occur once by chance in 1000 simultaneous studies addressing the same question)

Lyonisation — Inactivation of n-1 X chromosomes in an individual with n such chromosomes. Named after Mary Lyon, this mechanism ensures dosage compensation of genes encoded by the X chromosome. X chromosome inactivation does not occur in normal males who possess only one X chromosome but does occur in one of the two

X chromosomes of normal females. In males, however, who possess more than one X chromosome (i.e. XXY, XXXY, etc. individuals), the rule is the same and only one X chromosome remains active. X-inactivation occurs in early embryonic development and is random in each cell. The inactivation pattern in each cell is faithfully maintained in all daughter cells. Females are thus genetic mosaics, in that they possess two populations of cells with respect to the X chromosome: one population has one X active, while in the other population the other X is active. This is relevant to the expression of X-linked disease in females

Meiosis Cell division occurring in germ cells of sexually reproducing organisms, whereby gametes containing the haploid number of chromosomes are produced from diploid cells. Meiosis occurs in two phases, I and II: the reduction in number occurs during meiosis I

Mendelian Single gene disorder

Messenger RNA (mRNA) Template for protein synthesis. Genetic information flows: DNA→RNA→Protein

Missense mutation Single base substitution resulting in a codon for a different amino acid

Mitochondrial DNA DNA in the circular chromosome of mitochondria. Mitochondrial DNA is present in multiple copies per cell and mutates more rapidly than genomic (i.e. nuclear) DNA

Mitosis Cell division occurring in somatic cells, resulting in two daughter cells genetically identical to the parent cell

Monosomy Absence of one of a pair of chromosomes (e.g. monosomy X is Turner syndrome, 45XO)

Monozygotic Arising from a single zygote or fertilised egg. Monozygotic twins are genetically identical

Mosaicism Presence of two or more genetically distinct cell lines in the same individual, all arising from the same zygote

Multifactorial inheritance	Resulting from complex interplay of genetic and environmental factors
Mutation	Any heritable change in DNA sequence
Non-disjunction	Failure of two homologous chromosomes to disjoin during meiosis I, or two chromatids of a chromosome to separate in meiosis II or mitosis. The result is that both are transmitted to one daughter cell, while the other receives neither
Non-penetrance	Failure of expression of a phenotype in the presence of the relevant genotype
Nonsense mutation	Single base substitution resulting in the creation of a stop codon
Northern blot	Hybridisation of nucleic acid to immobilised RNA, so called in order to differentiate it from Southern blotting which was described first. Neither has any relationship to points on the compass
Obligate heterozygote (obligate carrier)	Individual who, on the basis of pedigree analysis, must carry the mutant allele
Oncogenes	Genes that, when overexpressed, result in neoplasia, in contrast to tumour suppressor genes which result in tumourigenesis when their activity is reduced
p	Short arm of a chromosome (from the French *petit*)
Palindromic sequence	DNA sequence that contains the same 5′ to 3′ sequence on both strands. Most restriction enzymes recognise palindromic sequences
Pedigree	Schematic for family with genetic disease, indicating relationships to the proband and affectedness with respect to the disease under consideration
Penetrance	All-or-none phenomenon related to the expression or otherwise of a disease in those individuals known to carry the relevant genetic mutation. In dominant disorders, this is the proportion of individuals known to be carriers (heterozygotes) who actually manifest the phenotype. Note the difference between penetrance and variable expressivity

Phenotype — Observed disease, abnormality or trait. An all embracing term that does not necessarily imply pathology. May be the result of genes, the environment or both

Pleiotropy — Diverse effects of a single gene on many organ systems (e.g. deficiency of the FBN 1 gene in Marfan's syndrome resulting in lens dislocation, aortic root dilatation, etc.)

Point mutation — Single base substitution

Polygenic diseases — Resulting from the interaction of many genes, some or all with minor effect (e.g. diabetes)

Polymerase chain reaction (PCR) — Molecular technique for amplifying DNA sequences. It is based on an iterative process of copying DNA and has become a standard technique in molecular biology research as well as routine diagnostics

Polymorphism — The presence in a population of two or more distinct variants, such that the frequency of the rarest is at least 1%. May be applied to phenotype or genotype. A genetic locus is polymorphic if its sequence exists in at least two forms in the population

Proband (propositus) — Index case. The affected individual through which the pedigree is ascertained

Probe — General term for a molecule used to make a measurement. In practice in molecular biology, a probe is a labelled DNA or RNA sequence used to detect its complementary sequence in a complex mix of sequences (e.g. in Southern blotting)

Pseudogene — Near copies of true genes. Pseudogenes share sequence homology with true genes but are inactive as a result of multiple mutations over evolutionary time

q — Long arm of a chromosome

Recessive — A recessive trait/disease is manifest only in homozygotes. For the X chromosome, recessivity applies to males who carry only one (mutant) allele. Females who carry X-linked mutations are generally heterozygotes and, barring unfortunate X-inactivation, do not manifest X-linked recessive phenotypes

Reciprocal translocation Exchange of material between two non-homologous chromosomes

Recombination Creation of new combinations of linked genes as a result of crossing over at meiosis

Recurrence risk Chance of recurrence of genetic disorder in a relative of an affected individual

Restriction enzymes Endonucleases from bacteria that cleave double-stranded (ds) DNA only at specific sequences. Named after the host restriction modification system found in bacteria, these are fundamental tools in molecular biology and diagnostics. Bacteria protect themselves from invasion of foreign DNA by producing restriction enzymes that will cleave foreign DNA at specific sites, rendering it functionless. The bacteria themselves protect their own DNA at the same sites by modifying the DNA using methylation (which protects the DNA from cleavage). Thus, for every restriction enzyme, it is likely that a corresponding methylase exists, although in practice only a relatively small number of these have been isolated

Restriction fragment length polymorphism (RFLP) DNA sequence based polymorphism that results in the creation of new restriction enzyme size fragments. Most commonly the polymorphism is a single base substitution, but may also be based on variation in length of a DNA sequence such as arises from variable number tandem repeats (VNTRs)

Restriction map DNA sequence map, indicating the position of restriction sites

Reverse genetics Identification of the causative gene for a disorder, based purely on molecular genetic techniques, when no knowledge of the function of the gene exists (the case for most genetic disorders)

Reverse transcriptase Enzymes that catalyse the synthesis of DNA on an RNA template. Contradicted the central dogma of genetics (DNA→RNA→Protein) and earned those who identified it the Nobel Prize in 1975

Ring chromosome Circular molecule resulting from deletion of material at both ends of the chromosome and subsequent reattachment of the ends

RNA (ribonucleic acid) Molecule containing ribose instead of deoxyribose (which occurs in DNA), into which DNA is transcribed

Robertsonian translocation Translocation between two acrocentric chromosomes, resulting from centric fusion. The short arms and satellites are lost

Sex chromosomes X and Y

Sibship All the siblings in a family

Silent mutation One that has no (apparent) phenotypic effect

Single gene disorder Disorder resulting from mutation at a single gene

Southern blot Method for transferring DNA fragments onto a solid support, such as a nitrocellulose filter. Hybridisation with a labelled probe can then be used to identify sequences immobilised in this way. Named after Ed Southern (currently Professor of Biochemistry at Oxford University, UK), the technique has spawned the nomenclature for other types of blot (Northern blots for RNA and Western blots for proteins)

Splicing Removal of introns from precursor RNA, in the generation of mRNA

Telomeres Ends of chromosomes

Teratogen Agent that increases the likelihood of congenital malformations (e.g. thalidomide)

Termination (stop) codon UAG, UAA or UGA. All cause termination of protein synthesis

Transcription Synthesis of ssRNA from a dsDNA template

Transfer RNA (tRNA) RNA molecules attached to the amino acid specified by the codon for which the tRNA carries the anticodon. Used for protein synthesis

Translation Protein synthesis directed by a specific mRNA

Translocation Exchange of chromosomal material between two or more chromosomes

Trisomy Three copies of a particular chromosome, instead of two

Unequal crossing over Occurs between similar sequences on chromosomes that are not properly aligned. Common where chromosome specific repeats are found and the basis of many microdeletion/microduplication syndromes

Variable expressivity	Variable expression of a phenotype. Not all-or-none (as is the case with penetrance). Individuals with identical mutations may manifest variable severity (e.g. monozygotic twins with Gerstmann-Straussler syndrome)
Western blot	Like a Southern blot but for proteins
X-autosome translocation	Translocation between the X chromosome and an autosome
X-chromosome inactivation	see Lyonisation